*Never Diet Again is about SIMPLE changes that will m
health. It takes a holistic view not just focusing on
but a wider approach looking at your sleep pattern, wate
helped me not to just get fit, but to get healthier!*
Georgie Muggleton – Dietician

*Never Diet Again is about truly adding value to a person's health for the long term, not a 5
minute feel good, quick fix health strategy. It has helped me improve my water consumption,
eat more regularly with the right foods and remove stimulants from my being. I have finally
found a health improvement program that works long term with the right values!*
Bruce Campbell – Awarded Number 1 Business Coach Globally

*Never Diet Again is not the quick fix promised by all the failed programs that my family and I have
tried over the years. But if you follow the well structured, often humorous lessons in the book; it
will be last program you will ever need to try. Why? Simply because it works. Following Never Diet
Again helped me lose 45kg in 12 months and I have never felt better or been healthier. My weight,
cholesterol and blood pressure are all down, and my vitality has skyrocketed. If you need direction
and guidance (and let's face it, we all do), it will change your life just as it has changed mine.*
Ivan Tyson – Businessman, Family Man and now Ironman

*Never Diet Again was a change of lifestyle challenge for us! We embarked on a journey to alter
the way we were living our everyday lives. From nutrition to exercise, each chapter gave us a new
perspective of how to attain the goals that we had set for ourselves when we started. This has been a
very worthwhile journey and has been carried on long after the completion of Never Diet Again.*
Barbara & Ted Wilkes – Retired

*I started Never Diet Again because I knew that if I didn't do something to become fitter,
I wouldn't be able to survive working the 90+hrs a week that I was. Call me cynical,
but when I started Never Diet Again, I did it with rolling eyes, and much complaining &
whining. Surprisingly, it wasn't many chapters in that I had a breakthrough, followed by
another and another. This book is a journey which allowed me many breakthroughs and in
the process, learn about myself, my body and my mind.*
Jo Murray – Restauranteur

*This is not just a book, this is a magical journey of the body and the spirit. All throughout
which we learn about ourselves and are gently nudged, closer and closer to the edge of the
nest, where we eventually leap out and immediately begin to soar, like the majestic creatures
Sharny and Julius allow us to come to realise we are. If you feel you are not living your life to
its full potential; buy this book and devour it immediately. It will change your life forever.*
Mark Jensen - Rugby League player and Businessman

Other titles by **sharnyandjulius™**

FITlosophy 1: Chasing Physical Perfection in a World of Gluttony
Where Have All The Pixies Gone?

Coming Soon to the collection:

FITlosophy 2: embracing excellence in a world of mediocrity

Pregfit: Preparing your body for a natural empowering birth

Beefed Up: Easily pack on muscle mass without steroids

The Athletic Pyramid: The science behind the magic

Never
DIET
Again

Escape the diet trap forever

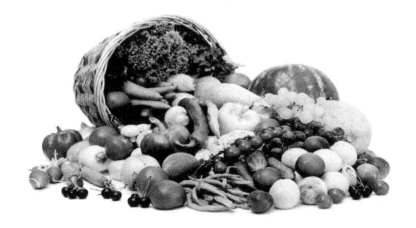

Never Diet Again by **sharnyandjulius**™
Escape the Diet Trap Forever

PO Box 7527
Sippy Downs
QLD 4556
Australia

ABN: 48 016 758 265
www.sharnyandjulius.com
email:info@sharnyandjulius.com

Edited: Glynny Kieser

Distributor: berminghambooks.com

Cover Photography: Steven Tyson

Typesetting and Design: Freshly Squeezed Design

Printed and bound in Australia

ISBN: 978-0-9871428-4-9

Dedication

This book is dedicated to Gwonny.

You showed us that to live a satisfied life, we need simply to ignore the inherent pessimism of our world, refusing to ever succumb to or even entertain the inevitable, unquestionable weakness of the mind and the most horrible of all phrases one could utter.

"I Quit."

For to give up allows all that is weak and worthless in this world to win, cloaking the amazing that every human spirit has to offer, the amazing that is only just around the corner from the current, seemingly impossible task.

For the impossible in life is merely a test, a lock to be picked, a puzzle to be solved – beyond which, personal fulfilment and satisfaction unimaginable by most is waiting to be danced with.

IMPORTANT!

BEFORE YOU BEGIN:

Go to:

www.sharnyandjulius.com/members

to register your copy of *Never Diet Again*
and get INSTANT ACCESS to over
$270 worth of FREE training.

Contents

Preface

Diets suck. We have seen far too many people spend money and time on diets, only to have their body image dreams shattered, leaving them fatter and more unhappy than before.

The world is changing and people are getting smarter. We now know that the "secret" to lasting fat loss is not going to be found in an ab machine or a shake. I mean seriously!! Do you want to be drinking shakes for the rest of your life? Is that the future you want to share with your kids, the whole family getting a liquid meal that tastes only vaguely like a chemicalised strawberry, chocolate or vanilla?

Cheat days, there's another diet myth we have found to be just clever marketing. Do you think quit smoking programs allow a cheat day? What about alcoholics anonymous? Do they prescribe a cheat day?

Unfortunately, people have been fooled, and sadly will continue to be fooled by the next gimmick promising the perfect body if they can only pull themselves away from their slobbery for just 2 minutes a day.

The new reality is that the people who take charge and responsibility for their own health and wellbeing are the ones who are going to win, the people who learn to listen to their bodies, before they listen to the advice of someone else. Trusting the innate knowledge of your own perfect body is the key to success in life, which begins with health.

Part of the problem is that there are so many conflicting diets.

There was a time in our lives where both of us were suffering through the heartache of being overweight and following the rollercoaster ride of working our way through all the major diet programs and books only to find failure and a further drop in self confidence at the end of each.

After failing many times and exhausting all of our options, we realised that the answers were not going to be found in these well marketed prescription diets. What we needed was education, and more importantly experience. We needed to learn about the human body, and more specifically our bodies, so we set out on a journey to find a way to never diet again.

After many years of learning and research, we put together the principles in this book, and decided to put them into practice. From that day on, using the simple lessons we had learnt, we managed to find a grander connection and vibrancy in our lives, we no longer let food control our lives, we no longer stressed about food, we no longer comfort ate, we no longer dieted. We were no longer passengers in our lives. We were (and still are) in control.

Once we had mastered our own lives, we put together a program called *Never Diet Again*, a weekly step by step blueprint to unlocking the secrets of your own body, and the way it interacts with the environment, nutrition and exercise. This program has been given to over a thousand of our personal training clients, and has changed their lives and countless more, for a healthier more confident person affects more than their own life. An inspirational person gives permission to others to be inspirational too.

Just think for a moment about how you could change the world if you could inspire 10 people around you to inspire 10 people around them... and it doesn't take any more effort, or sacrifice; it takes a little education, and a lot of trust in yourself.

The program has been going for over 3 years now, and the successes we have seen have been staggering. We've got graduates who have lost upwards of 50 kilos and kept it off, we have had previously couch bound graduates run marathons and ultramarathons, we've had people cured of high blood pressure, diabetes and heart conditions.

We've had marriages blossom into real, loving relationships and we've had families completely transform.

Most importantly, we have seen the true power of the human spirit emerge from people who were previously overburdened by self pity and self doubt. We have been privileged to witness the growth of some amazing leaders, parents, husbands, wives, daughters and sons.

We have witnessed the birth of inspiration.

It wasn't until last year that one of our clients asked us if there was a more cost effective way of delivering our program, as he felt that it would impact so well on his sister's family – they just couldn't afford the $2,700 tuition fee.

Imagine a world where you didn't have to suffer the pain of dieting. Dieting wasn't even a word you could relate to. Imagine going to a personal trainer or a gym to share the love of exercise, not to help you lose weight. Take a moment to imagine what wonderful things you could do with your life if you never had to worry about weight loss. How inspirational could you be?

This is the world we dream about every day. A world where the words "diet" and "weight loss" don't exist. A world where clothes are for keeping us warm and accentuating our individual beauty, not for hiding body fat.

This book is our way of helping a greater number of people to realise this dream for themselves, it is the book form of the program. Read it, action it, share it, teach it. Please enjoy.

Please; be inspirational.

Sharny and Julius.

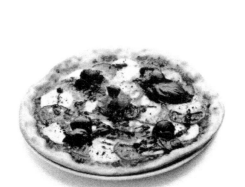

Why you're still fat ?

THIS book is probably not one of those books that you should read in one sitting. You could, it's nowhere near as long as the *Lord of the Rings*, but just reading it is not going to have as profound an effect on you as you were hoping, the lessons in it are to be explored, played with, experienced. Do that, and we guarantee that this book will change your life.

So, why is it that you are still fat? Well, we can break it down to 4 things.

You try to change too many things at once.

After years of eating what you want and avoiding exercise, you look at a photo of yourself and wonder how you got to be so sloppy looking. Like a bolt of lightning up your bum you realise that this has got to change. So you hire a personal trainer, or buy a diet program that promises to change your life.

On your first meeting, or when the package arrives, you are told to look at your current fat version of yourself, and then at a perfectly sculpted, good looking, tanned, hair free version of a perfect human body. Once you are feeling suitably uncomfortable, you are told that to get to this perfect physique, you will need to cut out all of your favourite foods, exercise like an Olympian every day, stop socialising, live like a mole and eat like a rabbit for the rest of your life.

Hey, you're pretty pumped, so at first this is doable. But after a month, a week, a day, or more often than not the first meal or first workout, it all becomes too much and you fail. Not completely, but cracks begin to show. You don't exercise as hard, or you sneak in a piece of chocolate...

Pretty sure you are smiling right now. Are you eating chocolate?

You focus on weight loss

This is the biggest problem with the easiest solution. Everything and everyone seems so obsessed with weight loss and weight gain. Your body is made up of so much more than just fat, in fact most of it is actually water. Your body's water content can fluctuate so much in one day depending on how much you drink, how much you have sweated, whether you have had coffee and what type of exercise you have done. More often than not, in the fad diets, the first week of weight loss is actually water loss. Water is stored in the muscles. Your muscles have gotten smaller. So now you look like a lighter, fatter, less energetic version of yourself. You still have all the fat, but less muscle.

But hey, you weigh less!

On this note, there are plenty of people who look thin who die of cancer and heart attacks every day. So what is the difference and what can you do?

Start focusing on being healthy. Fat loss is a side effect of being healthy (if you have fat to lose). Become a healthy person who eats good quality foods, exercises at a level that keeps your heart healthy, bones strong and muscles from degeneration. Throw the scales away, please!

You want instant results

If I told you that I had a pill that would strip your body fat down to 8% in 3 days, so you could be looking fantastic, how much would you pay for that?

Think about that amount of money, and how long it would take you to earn it. How many hours of hard work would it take to earn that kind of money, and why can't you spend that amount of time working on your body?

There is no magic pill that will make your body look perfect in a short time. What we love about fitness is that it is one of the only things on earth that is honest. There is no shortcut, there is only hard work. Nothing else. What you put in, you get out.

But that doesn't mean you can't be smart about it. The best shortcuts are through education, and knowing yourself. And this is what the book is all about.

Please understand this, the journey to great health is the fun part, nothing can prepare you for the elation you will feel when you buy new clothes every few months, because the ones you have are too big. Once you get to your healthy body, the adventures change to challenges.

"What can I do now?"

To get there is to strengthen your mind. Beyond that, you will have the mental toughness to tackle any physical challenge you want to put your body through.

You trust someone else with your greatest asset

Herein lies the greatest paradox to the human being.

You need other people to tell you about yourself.

We have become experts at analysing others, but are so afraid to analyse ourselves. Be it that we are afraid that we might find our weakness, or more likely, we are afraid that we might find the tiny twig that is holding back our inner greatness. We are so afraid that we might be amazing, that we enlist the help of others to tell us what is wrong with us. Justify our meagre existence.

Do you have a family member, a friend or work colleague who has issues that are so damn obvious to you, but you are amazed that they just don't see them. You really want to just slap them upside the head and say; "this is your problem, just fix it."

How frustrating are those people?

Now think about this; everyone you know is thinking that about you. It's human nature, we look for problems and flaws. Your friends are too afraid to look at themselves, so they find flaws in you. Take a moment to think to yourself, what is it that my friends think is a problem with me?

Now ask yourself how much better off you would be if you knew more about your body than your doctor, personal trainer, nutritionist, diet book, or health guru?

Well, that is exactly what this book is about. Through the lessons and tasks set out in this book, you will discover yourself; you will learn about your body's nuances. You won't need a doctor, you won't need a nutritionist, you won't need a diet book or a health guru. Leave those people to do the things that really matter like saving lives, rather than clog up their time with questions about losing weight.

Once you have read this book, and applied the lessons, we guarantee you will be a changed person, you will be educated, you will be confident. You will know yourself. You will never have to ask someone else about your body again. You will learn to look internally to find your answer, rather than look externally to find an excuse.

So let the learning commence, let's begin the discovery, let's unlock your secrets.

Your journey awaits.

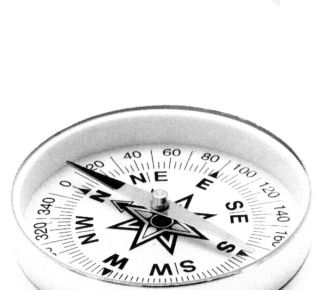

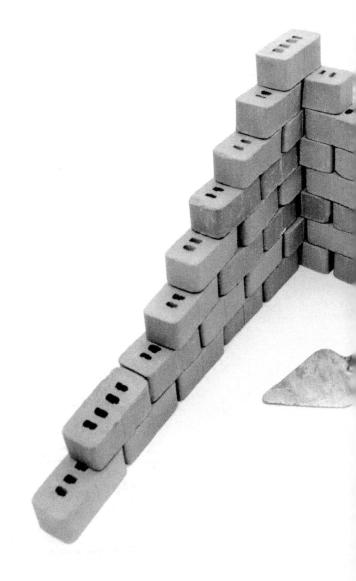

Part 1 – Foundations

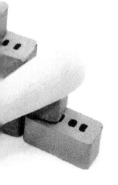

Change your thoughts and you change your world.

Norman Vincent Peale

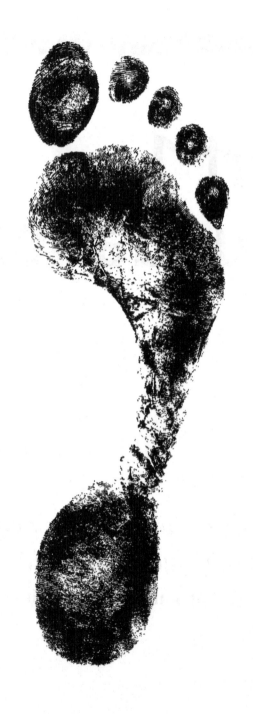

24

Degree Shift 1 - Track it

"A Journey of a thousand miles begins with just one step.

Confucious

BEFORE you can begin your journey, you need to map where you are currently. On the following pages you will find a food and exercise diary that will help you to see what areas of your eating and exercising need improving, and what areas you are excelling at.

The diary logs 7 days of eating and activity—and on the first page, we have provided an example for you to follow.

Each day is split into 5 sections.

Food — please log what you eat, when you eat it and the quantity. Please be honest, nobody is here to judge you—so don't hide anything. As far as quantity, be as accurate as you can, using measurements you can understand. If it is hard to judge, use the kitchen scale to measure the weight.

Sleep — please log the number of hours you slept, and the quality of your sleep (restless, deep, up and down, vivid dreams etc)

Exercise — please log your exercise completed here. If you have planned out activities for the week, put them in and when you have completed them, tick them off.

Water — please colour in the water bar to how much water you have drunk. Coffee and soft drinks do not count, just water.

Remember, one cup is 250ml, so 4 cups is a litre. This is the hardest to remember, so it's best if you fill it out every time you drink some.

Notes — any feelings or observations from the day.

Please complete this diary before commencing the next *Degree Shift*. If you do not, you will not get the full learning of the book before progressing onto the next level.

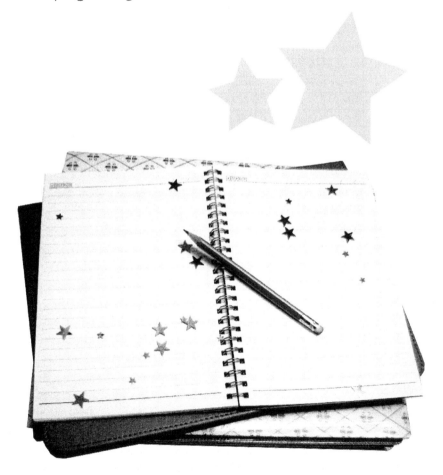

Date: 01/08/2011

Time	Food	Quantity
7am	Oats	1 cup
	Milk	1 cup
	Sugar	1 tbsp
8am	Orange	1
12:30pm	Pasta	1 cup
	Sauce	1/2 cup
	Cheese	100g
3pm	Rice biscuit (BBQ)	12
	Tuna (in spring water)	Small can
8pm	Steak	300g
	Roast potato (small)	4
	Roast pumpkin	200g
	Gravy	~1/3 cup
	Red wine (Merlot)	1/2 glass
8:30pm	Ice cream (Neapolitan)	1 bowl

Last night I slept for: 7 Hours

My sleep was: Broken

Exercise:

Walked dog for around half an hour before work.

Ran 5km at lunchtime at fast pace

Played tennis with Steve for 2 hours before dinner

Notes:

Felt really tired around 2pm

Water:

500ml	1 litre	1.5 litres	2 litres	2.5 litres	3 litres	3.5 litres	4 litres

Date: __/__/20__

Time	Food	Quantity

Last night I slept for: [   ] Hours

My sleep was: [   ]

Exercise:

Notes:

Water:

500ml	1 litre	1.5 litres	2 litres	2.5 litres	3 litres	3.5 litres	4 litres

Date: __ / __ /20__

Time	Food	Quantity

Last night I slept for: [ ] Hours

My sleep was: [   ]

Exercise:

Notes:

Water:

500ml	1 litre	1.5 litres	2 litres	2.5 litres	3 litres	3.5 litres	4 litres

Date: __ / __ /20__

Time	Food	Quantity

Last night I slept for: [   ] Hours

My sleep was: [   ]

Exercise:

Notes:

Water:

500ml	1 litre	1.5 litres	2 litres	2.5 litres	3 litres	3.5 litres	4 litres

Date: __ / __ /20__

Time	Food	Quantity

Last night I slept for: [   ] Hours

My sleep was: [   ]

Exercise:

Notes:

Water:

500ml	1 litre	1.5 litres	2 litres	2.5 litres	3 litres	3.5 litres	4 litres

Date: __ / __ /20__

Time	Food	Quantity

Last night I slept for: [   ] Hours

My sleep was: [   ]

Exercise:

Notes:

Water:

500ml	1 litre	1.5 litres	2 litres	2.5 litres	3 litres	3.5 litres	4 litres

Date: __ / __ /20__

Time	Food	Quantity

Last night I slept for: [ ] Hours

My sleep was: [   ]

Exercise:

Notes:

Water:

500ml	1 litre	1.5 litres	2 litres	2.5 litres	3 litres	3.5 litres	4 litres

34

Date: __ / __ /20__

Time	Food	Quantity

Last night I slept for: [ ] Hours

My sleep was: [   ]

Exercise:

Notes:

Water:

500ml	1 litre	1.5 litres	2 litres	2.5 litres	3 litres	3.5 litres	4 litres

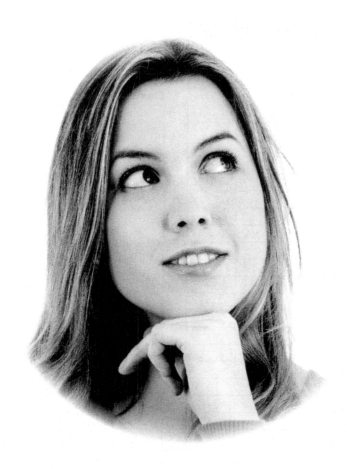

Degree Shift 2 – Dream

CONGRATULATIONS on completing your first task for *Never Diet Again*. **After a week of monitoring your eating, you should be feeling one of the following:**

- Excited and motivated

- Shocked, and a bit embarrassed

- Scared of what comes next

- Wondering what on earth *Never Diet Again* is all about.

I am sure that by the end of the week, you snuck in at least one "good" meal – one where you felt healthy, and were proud of it. That is great, and should be something that you hold onto.

Never Diet Again is not about instant fixes and whole of life changes. We see it all the time with the commercial diet plans and the shakes, and even the personal home goal of: "I'm going to go for a run every day" – too often the changes that are being affected are too far off your normal habits, that not long after, your body rejects them and you get demoralised – reverting back to old habits, and putting yourself under your own dark cloud of unhappiness.

Never Diet Again is about nudging you each week, just one more small degree in the right direction until you can live a sustainable, completely healthy life, and do it as a habit (easy), not out of willpower (difficult)!

This book is about only *one* shift at a time. Simple, manageable and permanent. On some of these shifts, you will see instant results, but the really exciting part is that the true benefits are for your future: playing sport into your 90s, completing events that you thought to never be possible, and *inspiring people around you.*

This not a get fit quick scheme. It is a progressive investment of time and effort into your health, leading to the ultimate destination: Life.

Life lived without constraints or excuses – whatever you can dream of is brought to possibility. Whatever you can conceive, you can do.

But before we do this, we need to have a *why*.

"Getting fit and losing weight" is a result. It is everybody's main goal when it comes to fitness. But "getting fit and losing weight" is not a tangible enough goal. How do you measure fitness, as it is relative to what you were yesterday? If you run today, but didn't run yesterday, then you are already fitter, and have achieved your goal? But then the benchmark has changed, since the goal is to get fitter, you need to do more tomorrow, and have therefore not reached your goal, and never will reach your goal – because you can always get fitter, no matter how fit you are.

This week, your task for *Degree Shift 2* is to create a tangible goal. Think of an event, one that you may have seen on TV, or heard about, or know of that requires physical endurance (fitness) to complete. Something that you "always wanted to do", something that you (or those around you) think is impossible in your current state. It doesn't even have to be a sporting event, it could be that you want to "fit into a size x dress", or "be off your diabetes medication".

These are the rules of the game if you want to pass this task and move onto *Degree Shift 3*:

- Fill in the boxes on the next page

- Your event has to be within the next 12 months.

- It has to be something that you or those around you don't think that you can do.

Remember, you don't need to tell anybody, you just need to write it in the book. Don't cut your goal in half because you think it's too bold – we believe in you, even if you don't.

My name is:	
My event is:	
The date my event is normally run:	
Who thinks I can't do it?	
Why I would like to do it:	

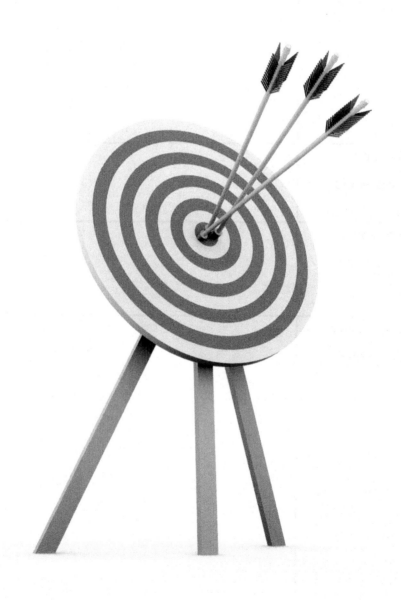

Degree Shift 3 – Goal

CONGRATULATIONS on creating a possibility for yourself. You should be feeling a little scared or a little silly at the thought of your dream. This is great, because it means that you are infinitely more likely to actually achieve it! Let us explain.

On a clear New Zealand winter day, a shy young boy named Ed called down quietly to his parents (Percy and Gertrude) from the elm tree that he was climbing in the back yard of his Tuakau home. He had gone up there to avoid conversation with the other boys who had come to his birthday party, and had been lost in his daydreams when he called out:

"Mum, Dad... One day I'm gonna stand on top of the world." On 29th May 1953 at the age of 33, Edmund Hillary and Tenzing Norgay became the first climbers to reach the summit of Mt Everest – the top of the world.

What a silly dream you think, but most of our best dreams were created as children, before society, looking good and consequence silenced them. But you have hopefully brought that to the surface – and that has taken some courage...

Now that you have dreamed your dream, it's time to make it real. This time, your task is to tell at least 5, but preferably 10 people what you are going to achieve. Don't worry about whether you think it is possible or not – you will deal with that in *Degree Shift 4*. The important thing is to tell as many people as you can about what you are going to achieve, and to tell them with conviction – so that they believe you.

On page 46 is space to fill in the names of the people that you spoke to, and their reactions.

To add a little more competition, you have three levels of conviction to your goal, the results of which will affect what happens in *Degree Shift 4*.

- Bronze: Tell 5 people

- Silver: Tell 10 people

- Gold: Tell as many people as you can to get 5 positive reactions and 5 negative reactions.

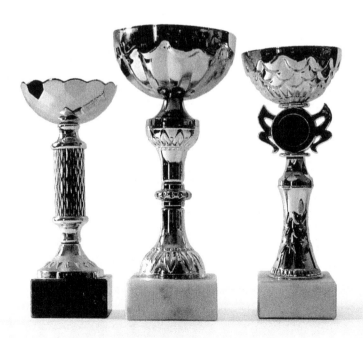

Name	Reaction
1	
2	
3	
4	
5	
6	
7	
8	
9	
10	
11	
12	

Degree Shift 4 – Alter Egos

CONGRATULATIONS on coming such a long way. You have created a powerful dream, turned it into a goal by giving it an expiry date, and you now have a cheer squad of at least 5 people!

You would have discovered through completion of *Degree Shift 3*, that if you tell the people around you with true conviction what your goal is; you will find it hard to find someone who has no faith in you. Can we therefore draw a conclusion that you are your greatest critic, not the people around you? If the people around you can believe in you, then why can you not believe in yourself?

If that is not a good enough question, try this:

"Why have you not already achieved your dream?"

Tell someone. Tell them right now. If there is nobody right next to you, go and find someone and tell them. This is important. Give them the two reasons that come into your head first. *Do not read any further until you have told them.*

Great, now that you have that off your chest – understand this: It is truly not your fault that you haven't yet achieved your dream. Entertain the idea that you might have multiple personality disorder...

> *"A dissociative mental disorder characterized by the existence in a person of two or more distinct, independent personalities"[1]*

Let's change *disorder* into *order* by identifying the problem. It's not *you* who has held you back, it's not *you* who makes you eat that cake, or drink that extra beer or put sugar into your coffee. It's not *you* who comes up with the excuses. It's not even *you* who is arguing in your head right now.

It's your alter ego. An alter ego (Latin, "the other I") is a second self, a second personality or persona within a person. It was coined in the early nineteenth century when schizophrenia was first described by early psychologists. A person with an alter ego is said to lead a double life.

[1] www.dictionary.com

Maybe we all do! Maybe you believe you have an angel and a devil on your shoulder – but I would argue that there is no angel telling you to do good things. It's just you. People are born good, not bad. That's why small children are so much fun to be around. They don't care about what others think. They just do what they want (dream) to do.

Somewhere along the line we develop the alter ego. And this alter ego is the person who sometimes takes over our lives and hushes our ambition with excuses. It's the voice inside your head that tells you that fat is OK, when deep down you want to be thin. Tells you that it's alright to be mediocre, when you want to shine like a star. Tells you to walk, when you want to feel the wind in your hair and the pulse in your throat.

It's the voice inside your head right now telling you that you don't have an alter ego. You're different to everybody else...

Tell it to shut up. "Shut up right now, I don't want your influence any more!"

It is said that the first step in solving a problem is to identify the source of the problem. The problem is that you have not achieved all that you want with your life. And the source is that you have an alter ego, who has held you back and prevented you from achieving your dreams.

Now some would say that identifying the problem is a solution in itself, but we will take it three steps further.

Step one: name your alter ego:

Step two: spend this week identifying the times where your alter ego takes over your life. Write them down if you like. Really pay attention to the arguments between you and your alter ego. Try to cut your alter ego short when it is attempting to lead you astray.

The point is to not beat yourself up any more – remember that you are perfect, just like a new born baby. All the things you are proud of are you, all the things you are not – belong to your alter ego.

Step three: Take a photo of yourself, print it out and mail it to us after you have written your alter ego's name on the back. Once it gets to us, we will look after it, and make sure that it gets the punishment that it deserves for holding you back for so long, while you go back into the world, uninhibited and infinitely powerful.

My alter-ego

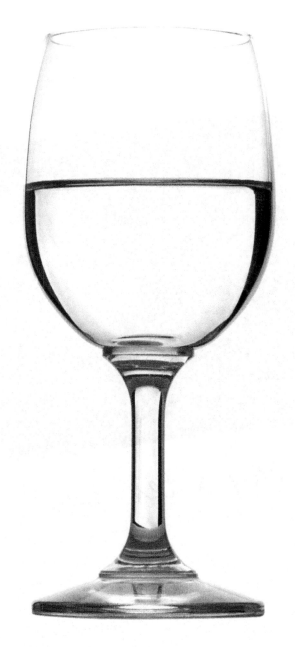

52

Degree Shift 5 – Drink more water 'til you got clear wee

We all know that water is good for us, but often the reasons are a little fuzzy. And even if we know why we should drink water, it's not a habit that many people form. But there are some very powerful reasons to drink lots of water every day, and forming the habit isn't hard, with a little focus.

Weight loss. Water is one of the most powerful weight loss tools, because it can replace high-calorie drinks like soft drinks, juice and alcohol. Water is a great appetite suppressant, and often when we think we're hungry, we're actually just thirsty. Water has no fat, no calories, no carbohydrates, and no sugar.

Heart healthy. Drinking a good amount of water could lower your risks of a heart attack. A six-year study published in the Journal of Epidemiology found that those who drink more than 5 glasses of water a day were 41% less likely to die from a heart attack during the study period than those who drank less than two glasses.

Cancer risk. Drinking a healthy amount of water has been found to reduce the risk of colon cancer by 45% and bladder cancer by 50% and potentially reduce the risk of breast cancer.

Energy. Being dehydrated can sap your energy and make you feel tired – even mild dehydration of as little as 1 or 2 percent of your body weight. If you're thirsty, you're already dehydrated – and this can lead to fatigue, muscle weakness, dizziness and even fainting.

Headache cure. Another symptom of dehydration is headaches. In fact, most headaches can simply be a matter of not drinking enough water.

Healthy skin. Drinking water can clear up your skin and people often report a healthy glow after drinking water. It won't happen overnight, but just a week of drinking a healthy amount of water can have noticeable effects on your skin.

Cleansing. Water is used by the body to help flush out toxins and waste products.

Digestive problems. Our digestive systems need a good amount of water to digest food properly. Often water can help cure stomach acid problems, and water along with fibre can cure constipation (often a result of dehydration).

Better exercise. Being dehydrated can severely hamper your athletic activities, slowing you down and making it harder to perform at your peak. Exercise requires additional water, so be sure to hydrate before, during and after exercise.

How to form the water habit

- **How much water?** It is not good to just drink when you're thirsty – you're already dehydrated by then. Form a routine by drinking a glass when you wake up, a glass before each meal, a glass in between meals, and be sure to drink before, during and after exercise. Try to keep yourself from feeling thirsty, and ensure that you have a long clear wee. (this means drink a minimum of 2 litres per day)

- **Carry a bottle.** A lot of people find it useful to keep a bottle of water at their desk, and drink from it throughout the day. When it's empty, fill it up again, and keep drinking.

- **Set a reminder.** Set your watch to beep at the top of each hour, or set a periodic computer reminder, so that you don't forget to drink water.

- **Substitute water.** If you would normally get a soft drink, or an alcoholic beverage, get a glass of water instead. Try sparkling water instead of alcohol at social functions.

- **Filter.** Instead of spending a fortune on bottled water, invest in a filter for your home. It'll make tap water taste like bottled, at a fraction of the price.

- **Exercise.** Exercising can help make you want to drink water more. It's not necessary to drink sports drinks like Gatorade or Powerade when you exercise, unless you are doing it for more than an hour. Just drink water. If you're going to exercise, be sure to drink water a couple hours ahead of time, so that it will get through your system in time, and again, drink during and after exercise as well.

- **Track it.** It often helps, when forming a new habit, to keep track of it – it increases awareness and helps you ensure that you're staying on track. Simply colour in the following bar chart to track your drinking this week, and be sure to drink at least 2 litres per day.

	Day1	Day2	Day3	Day4	Day5	Day6	Day7
4.0 l							
3.5 l							
3.0 l							
2.5 l							
2.0 l							
1.5 l							
1.0 l							
0.5 l							

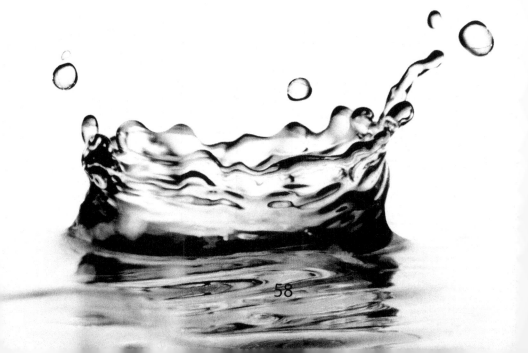

58

Degree Shift 6 - Superhydration

PLEASE re-read this before you go to bed tonight and again in the morning. Last week, you created the habit of regularly drinking water to ensure a healthier life. This week, we will take it a step further, by becoming more aware of your body through super-hydration.

Your brain controls your body, and is the receptacle of all of your feelings, so by dehydrating it, you essentially desensitise your feelings. Dehydration is therefore a state of numbness. By super-hydrating your body, you will become more sensorially aware. Simply, you will "feel" more.

Now put your philosophical hat on, and ponder the word "feel" in the following two sentences:

"I feel pain."

"I feel tired (sleepy)."

"Feel" has two different meanings? When you feel pain, it is a tactile sensation, whereas tired is an emotional sensation – completely different, or exactly the same?

Let's explore: When you feel tired, where do you feel it? It might help to point to the place(s) that you feel tired. (Generally your eyes, feet, head etc). If you do this exercise properly, you will notice that to feel tired is in fact a combination of tactile sensations. Try it with any emotion: Sad, happy, angry, love. As you "feel" them, try to point out where in your body those feelings are "felt".

This week, you will heighten your sensory perception to what it should be by super-hydrating your body. Then, you will simply observe your body as it "feels".

You need to be observant, and listen to your body – you will begin to see a side of you that you might not recognise. You will do things that will surprise you; so please pay attention to those things, and make note of them. So, to break it down into steps:

- I drank on average ____ litres of water a day last week

- I need to drink at least ____ litres of water a day this week (an extra litre a day)

- I will observe my feelings (physical and emotional), and make notes

If you think you are peeing too much, you are on the right track (average one wee per hour).

Specific things you might like to take note of:

- motivation levels

- concentration span

- general mood

- exercise

- recovery

- sleep

- general health (if you usually have pain somewhere, observe the levels this week)

- eating, specifically how you feel after you eat certain foods

- the effects of your usual pick me ups (coffee, tea, etc) and whether you actually need them

- anything else you feel is of note.

Take note of anything different, some people see colours brighter, others insist on having the window down when they drive because they like to feel the freshness of the air in their lungs, while some others just feel the urge to go for a run or walk, because it just "feels" perfect.

The following table should help you track your water consumption.

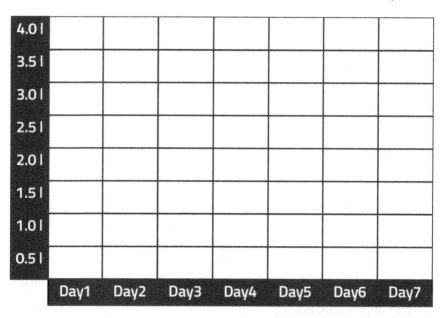

	Day1	Day2	Day3	Day4	Day5	Day6	Day7
4.0 l							
3.5 l							
3.0 l							
2.5 l							
2.0 l							
1.5 l							
1.0 l							
0.5 l							

Enjoy listening to your body as it explores its new possibilities, and you begin to understand the phrase "I feel alive!"

Degree Shift 7 – Micronutrients

THE most important step after adequate hydration is to ensure that you are nourished on a micronutrient[1] level. After completing the superhydration exercise, you would have begun to 'feel' your body's language as it talks to you. You may have noticed more strongly your cravings (did you crave something salty?). You are probably of the understanding that cravings are what make you unhealthy. Try changing your mindset to: "misreading your cravings is what makes your decisions unhealthy."

For example, when you superhydrate, your body expels the excess water, but along with it, it expels a lot of sodium which the body then tells you to replace by making you crave salt.

Misreading this to mean more than it does is what makes an unhealthy decision – I am craving salty chips. Your body will

---

[1.] A substance that an organism requires for normal growth and development but only in very small quantities, e.g. a vitamin or mineral associate what it needs (salt) with what it remembers getting it in its highest concentration (salty chips). There are much healthier ways of getting sodium.

But before you go throwing heaps of salt down your throat, we will correct any **micronutrient** imbalances before they occur – thus eliminating many common cravings.

If you eat only fresh produce and a variety of fresh meats and seeds every day, as well as gain exposure to adequate sunlight and get sufficient rest - you will be very close to being in balance. Unfortunately, not everybody can live this life - as we are time poor. The priorities of life dictate that you like to take shortcuts on nutrition so that you can focus on what is really important to you.

Fortunately for us, there is a shortcut to micronutrient balancing – multivitamin tablets. Before we can even look at your diet, we need to eliminate most potential "slip-ups" caused by getting many cravings in the first place.

A good multivitamin will help maintain strong bones, support immune system defences with a balance of essential antioxidants, help support energy production as well as proper muscle and nerve functions.

This time, please go to your chemist or supermarket and purchase a packet of once-a-day multivitamin/multimineral tablets. **Please read the health and allergy warnings. As with any supplement, if you are pregnant, nursing, or taking medication, consult your doctor before use.**

Take one tablet every morning before you eat your first meal, with your first glass of water.   Make sure that you continue to hydrate adequately (**until your wee is clear**), but listen to your body, if you feel thirsty, you are already dehydrated.

Please fill in the following chart, and jot your observations to move on to the next step.

Multivitamin brand chosen:

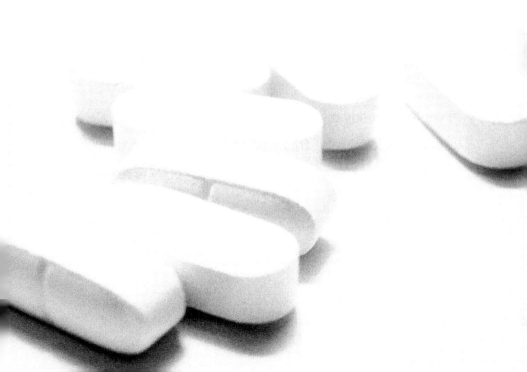

Day	Tablet taken	Observations
1	Yes / No	
2	Yes / No	
3	Yes / No	
4	Yes / No	
5	Yes / No	
6	Yes / No	
7	Yes / No	

If you are already taking a multivitamin tablet or you already eat a balanced diet, take this week to notice your cravings (if you have any), and try to work out what your body is really craving.

Degree Shift 8 –

Your eyes are bigger than your stomach

DO you ever get halfway through a meal and feel like you are full, but you continue to eat just so that you can clear your plate? Somewhere in the back of your head you have your grandmother's voice saying things like:

"If you don't finish what's on your plate,

you can't go out and play"

or

"Think about all the starving children in Africa."

Granny has a good point – why waste food? So instead of letting it go to waste, we let it go to waist... or hips, or butt, or thighs – maybe that flabby bit under the arms. After all, if the starving kids in Africa can't eat much, how better to empathise with them than to get fat by eating way past when we are full!

Having portion sized meals on a dinner plate makes them look small and unappealing. However, if you take the same portion and put it on a sideplate, it instantly looks bigger and more satisfying.

Eating off a small plate will allow you to control your portion size and not overeat. Overeating causes tiredness and bloating, as you overwhelm the body into lethargy. We are trying to get to a point where you are only eating what you need, and you are able to know *exactly* what your body *actually* needs.

This week, your task is simple. Eat all your meals off a sideplate, or out of a small bowl. That way, you won't be forced to eat more than you have to. Start by packing all your dinner plates away. Granny maths says you'll be saving hundreds of African kids a

68

day, and Grandpa will be happy that you are saving hundreds of dollars a month in food bills.

So to recap, you should be having a glass of water before every meal, and your meals should be served on a sideplate. Every morning, you should be having a multivitamin with a glass of water, and during the day, you will drink enough water to have long clear wee and to never feel thirsty. Simple really!

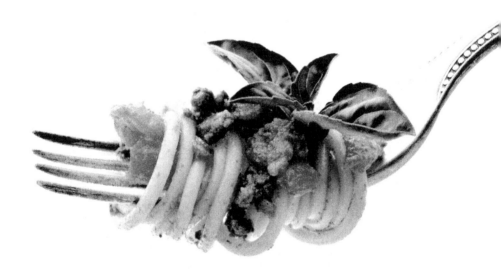

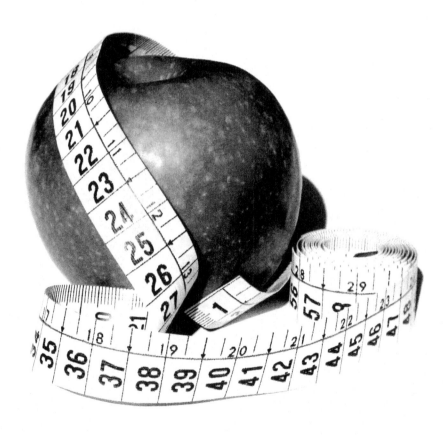

Degree Shift 9 –

Eat more frequently to burn more fat

BASAL METABOLIC RATE (BMR) is the amount of energy expended while at rest. This varies depending on body composition and genetics.

THERMIC EFFECT OF FOOD is the increase in energy expenditure above your BMR, due to the cost of processing food for storage and use.

So, you burn a certain amount of energy per day, just to stay alive. You also burn a certain amount of energy digesting your food. Good news – you don't have to feel guilty about eating – it's a requirement to stay alive.

In *Degree Shift 8*, you worked on eating smaller portions, as you now know that huge meals make you tired, and put your body into "storage mode." This week, you will be working on food timing – probably the most critical shifts in the entire journey to a healthier you.

When you eat is more important than *what* you eat. More specifically – how often you eat is a step that needs to be fixed before you can look at what you eat.

Now that you can consistently eat off a side plate, your goal is to eat 6 meals per day, spaced no more than 3 hours apart.

Eating 6 smaller meals a day will boost your metabolic rate (the amount of energy you burn in a day), due to the thermic effect of food. Eating more frequently means that you are burning more energy more often, which means that you are burning away your fat!

Another benefit is that your energy levels will stay on a consistent level, because you are maintaining balanced blood sugar levels, preventing hunger attacks.

You will also find it easier to build and maintain muscle. The more muscle you develop, the faster your metabolism becomes. Frequent meals help promote muscle growth by regulating insulin levels and providing a steady flow of amino acids into the muscle cells.

By eating approximately every three hours you are constantly delivering a steady output of insulin, which is necessary for muscle growth and glycogen storage.

Insulin plays a major role in transporting glucose and amino acids into the muscle cells where they can then be used for recovery and muscle growth.

Frequent meals also allow for more efficient use of vitamins and minerals. Your body simply becomes much more effective at processing these vital nutrients.

To reap the full benefit of this lifestyle, be sure that you eat on a consistent schedule. This requires a bit of meal planning, but it is certainly worth it. It is very important to get your body into the habit of knowing when it will be supplied with nutrients. This way, your body won't fall into dreaded hunger attacks and cravings. Instead, it will always know that a steady flow of nutrients will soon to be supplied.

By eating 5 to 6 small meals per day, you will increase your energy levels, accelerate muscle growth, and speed up your metabolism without storing fat.

Use the following table to chart your progress this week.

	Meal 1	Meal 2	Meal 3	Meal 4	Meal 5	Meal 6
Day 1	Time:	Time:	Time:	Time:	Time:	Time:
Day 2	Time:	Time:	Time:	Time:	Time:	Time:
Day 3	Time:	Time:	Time:	Time:	Time:	Time:
Day 4	Time:	Time:	Time:	Time:	Time:	Time:
Day 5	Time:	Time:	Time:	Time:	Time:	Time:
Day 6	Time:	Time:	Time:	Time:	Time:	Time:
Day 7	Time:	Time:	Time:	Time:	Time:	Time:

Remember:

- eat at least 6 meals per day

- do no leave more than 3 hours between meals

- snacks are counted as meals (fruit, muesli bars or protein shakes)

- meals must be less than a side plate in size

- eat your first meal as soon as you wake up, after your glass of water and multivitamin

- drink plenty of water

- enjoy feeling consistently healthy!

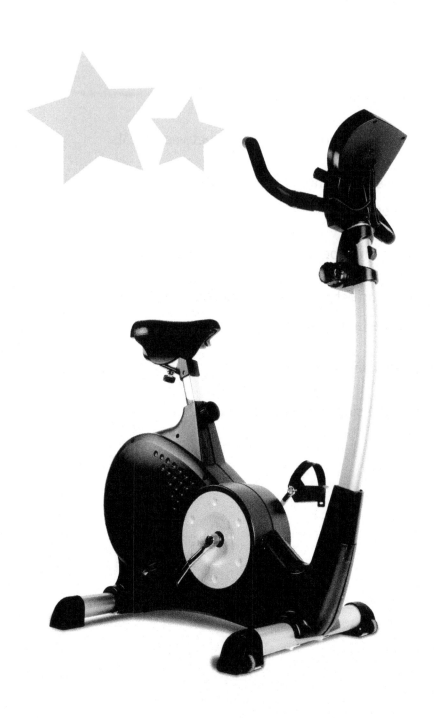

Degree Shift 10 – Finally, some huff and puff

Well done, you have now set up your basic nutrition routine, and should be feeling healthy, strong and more energised. There are two more areas to cover before you can move on to *Never Diet Again* Level 2; sleep and exercise.

By now you should be quite active. Please fill in the following table of what you plan to do this week for exercise. Include everything, be proud.

Day	Physical Activities
Monday	
Tuesday	
Wednesday	
Thursday	
Friday	
Saturday	
Sunday	

The government spent millions of dollars recommending it, you know you're meant to do it and we're prescribing it. 30 minutes of physical activity every day. At least. *Never Diet Again* is not about subscribing to normalcy. If the government says that you should do at least 30 minutes of physical activity every day to avoid obesity, we will agree that you are not obese and you don't want to just be normal, so this week, we will add 30 minutes of physical activity to what you normally do. Every day.

How to proceed to the next level:

- before you move, fill out what is normal for you to do (if you haven't already)

- do what you said you were going to do and tick off the activities as you do them

- during the week, in a different colour pen, describe your extra 30 minutes for each day

- have fun being active!

Degree Shift 11 - Sleep

SLEEP deprivation can result in the following problems: Iritability, memory lapses or loss, impaired moral judgement, severe yawning, hallucinations, symptoms similar to ADHD, impaired immune system, diabetes, increased heart rate variability, decreased reaction time and accuracy, tremors, aches, growth suppression, obesity and decreased temperature.

Studies have shown that oversleeping has been consistently associated with increased mortality.

Clearly, this is something we want to get right then? Too much and you die, too little and you may wish you were dead!

So how much sleep do we need? Babies need 18 hours a day, children anywhere between 9 and 15 hours, and teenagers need nearly 10 hours a day! Most studies show that an optimal amount of sleep for an adult is between 6 and 8 hours. A University of California study of more than one million adults found that those who live longest, are people who sleep 6-7 hours each night.

We are not going to tell you exactly how much sleep you need, just that it needs to be between 6 and 8 hours per night. No more. If you sleep too little, try to catch it up during the day with a cat nap – don't just have a huge sleep the next day. If you feel you are sleeping too little, just go to bed half an hour earlier - do not change your waking time as this affects your circadian rhythm (biological clock). Have you ever noticed that sleeping in actually makes you tired for that day?

This week, your task is to make quality sleep a priority. On page 85 is a sleep diary. It is important to fill it out every day, as you will be able to work out why you had the particular quality of sleep you had. Things you might want to try to ensure a quality sleep:

- If you feel tired, go to bed. Don't force yourself to stay up for that TV show. Just press record

- Do not drink caffeine or alcohol within 3 hours of going to bed

- Your bedroom should be cool

- Do not sleep immediately after eating (leave at least 2 hours)

- Avoid large, fatty or spicy dinners

- Shower before bed (if you don't already)

- Go to the toilet before you sleep

- Set an alarm

- Avoid sugars before bed (they raise insulin levels and force you to store fat)

- Exercise at least 30 minutes per day

- Resolve all arguments

- Write down the problem that is plaguing you (or the to-do list for tomorrow)

- Drink a cup of chamomile tea

- Try to sleep in complete darkness (notice how it is harder to sleep on a full moon?)

- Rotate your mattress every month, and replace it every 10 years

- Magnetic underlays do work

- Don't watch TV in bed – TV shows try to keep you stimulated

- Turn your phone off

- Stretch before bed

- Read a few pages of a book

- Orgasm just before bed (you don't need to write this one down)

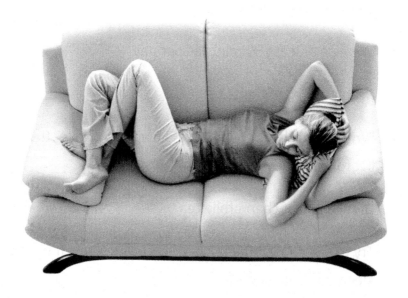

Day	Hours of sleep	Quality of sleep	Why do I think the quality of my sleep was what it was?

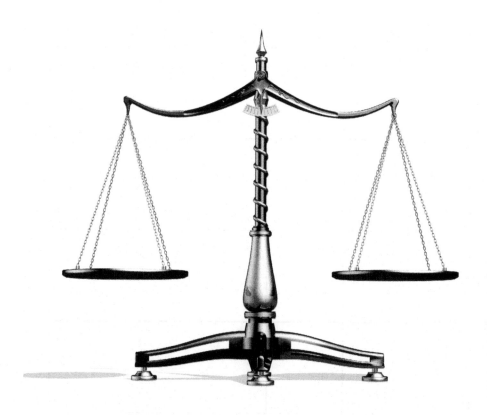

Degree Shift 12 - Compare

CONGRATULATIONS on completing all the preliminary steps in the *Never Diet Again – Foundations* course. Please fill out this food and exercise diary so that you can graduate to the next level (*Never Diet Again – Food Quality*), where you will learn all about the quality of the foods that you put into your body. This *is* a test; to pass, you must satisfy all the requirements to be a healthy individual, based on what you have learned. You have been following all the steps closely, so you should breeze through it with ease!

- Drink at least 2 litres of water every day (*Never Diet Again* 5)

- Take a multivitamin every morning (*Never Diet Again* 7)

- Eat off a sideplate (*Never Diet Again* 8)

- Eat 6 meals per day (*Never Diet Again* 9)

- Do not leave more than 3 hours between meals (*Never Diet Again* 9)

- Do at least 30 minutes of physical activity every day (*Never Diet Again* 10)

- Sleep between 6 and 8 hours per day—no more (*Never Diet Again* 11)

Date: __ / __ /20__

Time	Food	Quantity

Last night I slept for: [   ] Hours

My sleep was: [   ]

Exercise:

[   ]

Notes:

[   ]

Water:

500ml	1 litre	1.5 litres	2 litres	2.5 litres	3 litres	3.5 litres	4 litres

Date: __ / __ /20__

Time	Food	Quantity

Last night I slept for: [ ] Hours

My sleep was: [ ]

Exercise:

Notes:

Water:

500ml	1 litre	1.5 litres	2 litres	2.5 litres	3 litres	3.5 litres	4 litres

90

Date: __/__/20__

Time	Food	Quantity

Last night I slept for: [ ] Hours

My sleep was: [   ]

Exercise:

Notes:

Water:

500ml	1 litre	1.5 litres	2 litres	2.5 litres	3 litres	3.5 litres	4 litres

91

Date: __/__/20__

Time	Food	Quantity

Last night I slept for: [ ] Hours

My sleep was: [ ]

Exercise:

Notes:

Water:

500ml	1 litre	1.5 litres	2 litres	2.5 litres	3 litres	3.5 litres	4 litres

Date: __ / __ /20__

Time	Food	Quantity

Last night I slept for: [ ] Hours

My sleep was: [ ]

Exercise:

Notes:

Water:

500ml	1 litre	1.5 litres	2 litres	2.5 litres	3 litres	3.5 litres	4 litres

Date: __ / __ /20__

Time	Food	Quantity

Last night I slept for: [ ] Hours

My sleep was: [ ]

Exercise:

Notes:

Water:

500ml	1 litre	1.5 litres	2 litres	2.5 litres	3 litres	3.5 litres	4 litres

Date: __/__/20__

Time	Food	Quantity

Last night I slept for: [ ] Hours

My sleep was: [   ]

Exercise:

Notes:

Water:

500ml	1 litre	1.5 litres	2 litres	2.5 litres	3 litres	3.5 litres	4 litres

95

Before I started *Never Diet Again*, **my energy levels were (out of 10):**

1	2	3	4	5	6	7	8	9	10

<<Can't get out of bed   **Jumping for joy>>**

They are now at:

1	2	3	4	5	6	7	8	9	10

<<Can't get out of bed   **Jumping for joy>>**

The most important lessons I have learnt from Never Diet Again—Foundations:

The best step was:

My thoughts on Never Diet Again - Foundations:

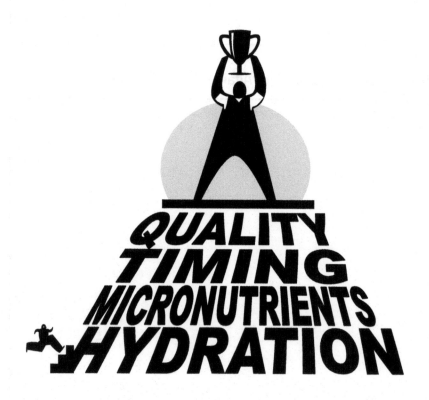

Completion Part 1 - Foundations

THANK you and congratulations on completing your food and exercise diary. To have come this far is a great achievement in itself and you deserve to be congratulated and to feel good about yourself.

Take some time to reflect on how far you have journeyed. Think about what you have learned and what decisions you make about your health now, based on the *Never Diet Again* education program.

As you have now progressed through all the steps to build a solid foundation of health, we can only now look at what you eat. Isn't it interesting that we have not touched on actual foods for more than 13 sessions?

By building the foundations, we have ensured that your results are permanent, and that they are based on education and your own experience. *Never Diet Again* – Food Quality will follow the same format – learning and experiencing for yourself one shift at a time, so that the lessons and experiences can have a lifelong impact.

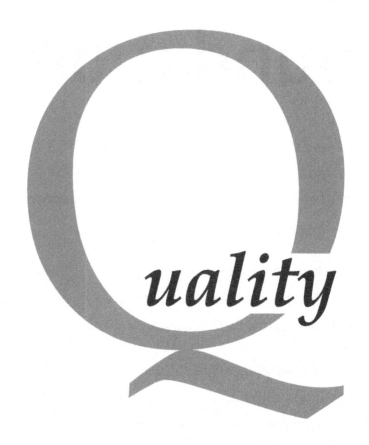

Part 2 – Food Quality

It is the quality of our work which will please God and not the quantity.

Gandhi

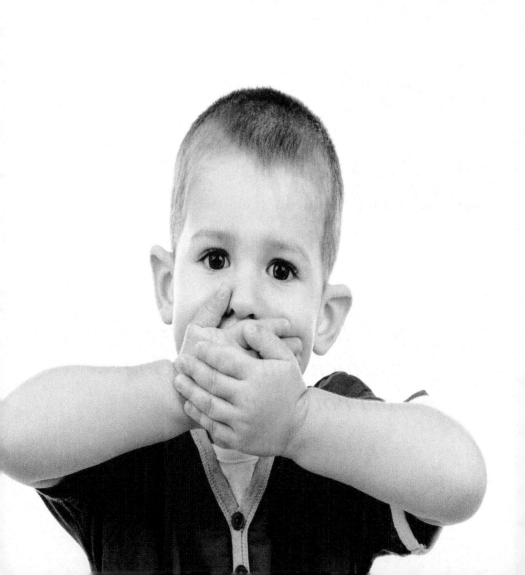

Degree Shift 13 – The C word

ONCE again, congratulations on completing the foundation course of *Never Diet Again*, and welcome to the second instalment – where you will be educated on the quality of certain foods, and will therefore be able to make informed decisions for your own health.

You've heard about them, you've probably counted them or monitored them or you've joked about them. The "C" word...

Calories

What is a Calorie? A calorie is a unit of measurement — but it doesn't measure weight or length. A calorie is a unit of energy. When you hear something contains 100 calories, it's a way of describing how much energy your body could get from eating or drinking it.

Some people watch their calories when they try to lose weight. This can be very tedious and time consuming, and focuses too much on food – remember that food is a fuel, and obsessing over it is unhealthy. For this chapter, however – we will delve into calories as a learning experience – so that we can understand them, and make informed decisions about them.

Your body is like a bank account. If you put in more money (food) than you can spend, you will save it (as fat). If you earn less money than you spend, then you will need to dip into your savings. So as your body's accountant, you could be telling yourself that it might be time to live a little, cut back the hours spent saving – maybe even go on a spending spree! But before we go starving ourselves and running a marathon, we need to work out if we are running at a profit, or a loss.

It is simple, really - Energy in vs. Energy out. If you put more energy into your body than you need for your day of living, then your body will store that energy (measured as calories) as fat. If you put less fuel into your body than you need – your body will burn some stored fat!

So what you need to do then, is calculate how much energy you consume in any given day (just add up the calories for the day), then take away how much energy your body uses for the day.

- **Calories in *equals* calories burnt (maintenance)**

- **Calories in *less* than calories burnt (fat loss)**

- **Calories in *more* than calories burnt (fat storage)**

Clearly, you want to be at maintenance or fat loss, unless you are preparing to hibernate or are a body builder. To calculate your daily calorific requirements, complete the following calculation:

Men:

Weight in kg: [ ]   multiply this by 13.7= [ ] =a

Height in cm: [ ]   multiply this by 5 = [ ] =b

Age in years: [ ]   multiply this by 6.8 = [ ] =c

66 + a + b − c = [ ] = BMR **(Basal Metabolic Rate)**

Women:

Weight in kg: [ ]   multiply this by 9.6= [ ] =a

Height in cm: [ ]   multiply this by 1.8 = [ ] =b

Age in years: [ ]   multiply this by 4.7 = [ ] =c

665+a+b−c= [ ] = BMR **(Basal Metabolic Rate)**

Now to calculate your Maintenance calories, simply multiply your BMR by an activity multiplier:

Sedentary = BMR x 1.2 (Little exercise, desk job)

Lightly Active =BMR x 1.375 (light exercise/ sports
1-3 days per week)

Moderately Active =BMR x 1.55 (moderate exercise/sports
3-5 days per week)

Very Active =BMR x 1.725 (hard exercise/sports
6-7 days per week)

I require _____ calories per day to maintain my current body weight. (calories out)

To calculate calories in, you simply look at the food labels. And for foods that don't have labels, there is a great free online resource called www.calorieking.com. Simply add up your calories for the day to see what your "calories in" equates to. Do this for one day this week.

I ate _____ calories in one day. (calories in)

Now calculate the difference:

calories in – calories out = _____

If your number above is positive, you are going to store fat. If you are around even, or slightly negative you are being healthy.

WARNING: Do not undercut your maintenance calories by more than 500 calories per day; otherwise you will go into starvation mode, which is dangerous for your body. Calorific deficit dieting only works if you have small deficits every day, and you do it consistently. Crash dieting is very dangerous.

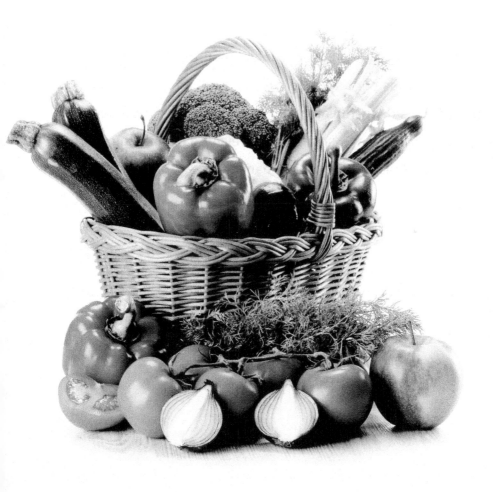

Degree Shift 14 – Macronutrients

OVER the next few chapters, you will be learning about the basic macronutrient food types, namely Carbohydrates, Proteins, Fats and Fibre. We will highlight the good, the bad and the ugly of each, so that you can make educated decisions as to what you will put into your body. Prescribed diets may well help people lose weight, but nutritionally educated people can wade through all the fads, and make their own decisions about what is right for them.

Every human body is unique, so why should everybody eat exactly the same? The framework may well be the same, but only you will know exactly what works for you. To get to that point however, takes trial and error, and the most efficient way through the trial and error process is with prior knowledge.

So sit down at your desk, clear your mind for some learning and hand your teacher an apple, because class is in session!

Carbohydrates are an important nutrient found in many foods. Examples of foods that contain carbohydrates include bread, breakfast cereal, rice, pasta, fruit, potato, corn, dried beans and lentils, sugar, milk and yoghurt.

Carbohydrate is an important source of energy for the body. The Dieticians Association of Australia (DAA) recommends you try and eat carbohydrate-containing foods in every meal to provide the body with energy throughout the day.

The rate at which carbohydrate-containing foods are digested varies greatly. The comparative rate at which the body receives energy from carbohydrates through digestion is called glycaemic index or GI – we will fully explain this concept in the following chapters.

Protein is an important nutrient used in the growth and repair of cells. Protein can come from animal or plant foods such as meat, chicken, fish, eggs, nuts, seeds, dried beans, lentils, dairy products or soy products.

Interestingly, protein can also be used for energy if enough carbohydrate foods are not eaten. Protein needs are increased during times of cell growth or repair, such as childhood and adolescence; pregnancy and lactation; during and after illness or surgery; and after strenuous exercise.

Fat is an essential part of our diet and is important for good health. There are different types of fats, with some fats being healthier than others. The DAA suggests that to help make sure you stay healthy, it is important to eat 'healthy' fats in moderation as part of a balanced diet. When we talk about fats in the following pages, we will cover all the types of fats in detail.

Fibre or dietary fibre is the part of food that is not digested in the small intestine. Rather, dietary fibre moves largely unchanged into the large intestine or colon where it is fermented by friendly bacteria that live there. Eating more dietary fibre can help to keep the digestive system healthy and reduce the risk of constipation, diverticular disease, haemorrhoids and bowel cancer.

Fibre can be soluble, insoluble or resistant starch. We will cover fibre in the following chapters.

So there you have it, lesson one – an overview of the food types. Over the following chapters, as you learn about these important nutrient types, you should begin to understand your food better. By the end of these next few chapters, you should be able to make accurate and educated decisions based on your own personal health and lifestyle goals.

In the meantime, start to think about what you already know, as knowing what you know (or more importantly knowing what you don't know – or even knowing that you don't know) will help you to learn about what you don't know and make it something that you do know, and do it quicker. Hopefully we will just be clarifying and revisiting what you already know!

Tiny little teaser: Whether that last paragraph made sense to you or not, has something to do with good fats... All will be revealed in time.

Degree Shift 15 - Carbohydrate

CARBOHYDRATE is an important nutrient found in many foods. Examples of foods that contain carbohydrate include bread, breakfast cereal, rice, pasta, fruit, potato, corn, dried beans and lentils, sugar, milk and yoghurt.

Carbohydrate is an important source of energy for the body. The Dieticians Association of Australia (DAA) suggests eating carbohydrate-containing foods in every meal to provide the body with energy throughout the day.

 To simplify it right down, carbohydrates are *any number* of molecules of sugar, joined together. The diagram to the left is a scientific model of a sugar molecule, like you used to make in science class, if you were paying attention.

Simple carbohydrates are 1 to 2 of these molecules joined together, and as you can imagine, are simple to digest. Examples of simple carbohydrates are glucose, fructose (the sweet taste in fruit) and table sugar (which is a glucose and fructose joined).

Complex Carbohydrates are 3 or more of these molecules joined together. The more sugar molecules joined together, and the more intricate the structure, the more complex, and therefore the harder it is to digest.

The rate at which carbohydrate-containing foods are digested varies greatly, depending on their complexity. The comparative rate at which the body receives energy from carbohydrates through digestion is called glycaemic index or GI.

So, a simple carbohydrate would have a high GI value, because it is easy to digest, and therefore turned into energy very fast in your body. This is why sports drinks are high in simple carbohydrate (sugar) – athletes need energy fast while they are on the run!

A very complex carbohydrate would have a low GI value – and would require a lot of work from your body to digest, and therefore provides a slow steady stream of energy, rather than a spike.

So, why should this matter, if all carbohydrates are turned into energy (through blood glucose) anyway? What's all the big fuss about?

Well, your body can only use a certain amount of energy: If you don't use the blood glucose, it gets stored. Luckily if you exercise, your body stores it as glycogen first (in your liver or muscles) but when you have full glycogen stores, there is only one option left! Fat.

Over the next 3 days, you have an experiment to conduct. Eat a low GI breakfast, a medium GI breakfast and a high GI breakfast (not all on the same day!), and see what happens to your body. Please try to eat the foods on an empty stomach and avoid coffee if at all possible. Record your results in the table on the next page (how fast you felt the energy, how long until you felt hungry again, and how your energy levels fluctuated.)

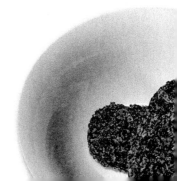

Food	GI level	Observations
White bread with honey or jam (no butter)	High	
Weetbix with milk	Medium	
Traditional Oats	Low	

Once you have completed the experiment, you will be able to make an educated decision on what types of carbohydrates to have and when, without having to rely on fad diets and experts. Fantastic!

Degree Shift 16 – Insulin

WE looked at the GI value of foods. To recap, simple carbohydrates will generally have a high GI – they will be digested very quickly, turned into blood glucose, and used as an energy source. If not, they are stored. Complex carbohydrates are harder to digest, and therefore release energy more slowly.

We also touched on Glycogen. **Glycogen** is the body's primary source of fuel when we do strenuous exercise. This is important to understand, as fat is used only when the body is not under stress, or when the glycogen levels have been nearly depleted. Glycogen is stored in the liver as well as the muscles.

When you do strenuous exercise, your liver and muscles release glycogen (stored energy) first. Not fat. When glycogen is released into the blood, it just so happens to be released as blood glucose, so that it can be used by the muscles that require it.

As you can imagine, thousands of years ago humans only ate meat from animals, roots and vegetables that they could gather – there was no such thing as refined sugar, or a sports drink. Glycogen would therefore have been a very important commodity for the human body (imagine running away from a lion – you would need energy pretty quickly, and would have some problems if you waited for your fat to be turned into energy – a very slow process). Glycogen gets turned into energy very quickly, as it is simply stored glucose.

Now, imagine those thousands of years ago; put your fur coat on, get your club and break out your inner caveman or cavewoman. Imagine how hard it would be to get carbohydrates. Even now, if you were dropped in the outback where there are no shops – how hard would it be to get carbohydrates?

Glycogen can only be stored if there is enough blood glucose. Blood glucose comes from carbohydrates, which are traditionally difficult to find – as a caveperson. So when you get chased by that lion, your body's glycogen stores release a flood of glucose into the blood. Once all the running is done and you are safe, you will still have some unused glucose floating around in your blood. Considering it was so hard to forage enough roots and vegetables to fill your glycogen stores, would it be wise to just cleanse the body of the unused glucose through urination, or to get it back into the muscles and liver as glycogen – in case that lion comes back?

This is where insulin comes into play. **Insulin** is a hormone in the body that triggers storage. When your blood glucose levels are high (after strenuous exercise), your body releases insulin to prevent you from losing any of it. Imagine insulin as a hoarder of blood glucose (and other molecules, such as protein and fat). When insulin is around, it just wants to put stuff into cells. Glycogen first – replace the survival stuff first, then if there is any more around, we need to store it as fat – don't let anything go to waste. Store, store, store. And when it is done storing, it hangs around in the blood, waiting to store more – just in case.

Now, fast forward to today. When we eat high GI foods, our body is flooded with glucose really quickly, the body thinks we have just run away from a lion, and releases a flood of insulin – "don't let any of that glucose go to waste!" If your glycogen stores are in fact low (after strenuous exercise), the insulin will ensure that they are replenished. Once your glycogen stores are full, insulin pushes glucose into the fat cells of the body. Store, store, store.

Once the storage is done, your insulin hangs around for up to 6 hours waiting for more to store. This is why you feel hungry very soon after a high GI meal, and stay hungry for up to 6 hours – and to top it off, you're hungry for more glucose - more high GI food, which starts the cycle again! Wonderful if you are a caveman, but treacherous if you have easy, unlimited access to high GI foods.

Because insulin is a storage hormone that stores anything, it can also be used advantageously or abused. For example, some bodybuilders inject synthetic insulin to ensure that their muscles store as much protein as possible (this is extremely dangerous). If you want to get protein or carbohydrates to your muscle fibres fast after a workout, an insulin spike will ensure that they get there fastest. Hence the sports drink after a big run, and why some protein drinks have added sugar.

Can you see why you would not drink a sports drink before a run? Because it would release an insulin spike before you exercise, making your body go into storage mode, retarding your performance as your body is fighting against itself. One half wanting to store the glucose, and the other half needing to use it!

But the biggest learning is that high levels of insulin, combined with high fat in your diet will make you store all the fat that you eat. Handy if you want to be a sumo wrestler!

So, your task for *Degree Shift 16* is to write down 3 foods or meals that you eat (or used to eat) that were a combination of high GI carbohydrates, and high fat.

| Sumo Food 1: |
| Sumo Food 2: |
| Sumo Food 3: |

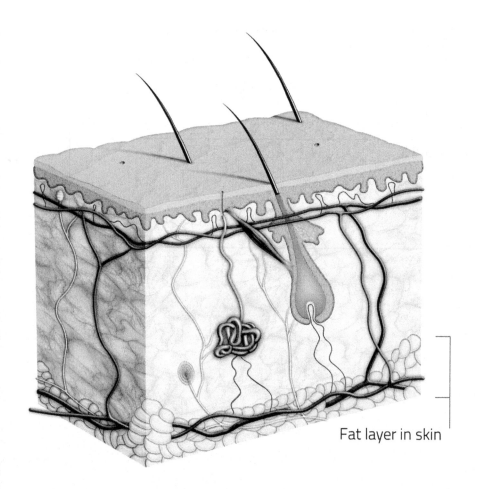

Fat layer in skin

Degree Shift 17 – Fat

NOW that you are an expert in *Carbohydrates, Glycaemic Index* and *Glycogen*, we can move on to learning about our next food group. Fats.

Before we delve into the different types of dietary fat, we need to first look at human body fat, and clarify some myths.

Fat Fact 1:

Fat is stored in what is called adipose tissue (fat cells). A fat cell (you have 50 billion of them) is just a storage cell. An empty bag (for thin people) or a bulging full bag (for fat people).

Fat Fact 2:

Adipose tissue can be found in the following places:

- In between muscles

- Packed around internal organs (visceral fat)

- Subcutaneously (under the skin – see diagram on page 122)

Fat Fact 3:

Female sex hormones cause fat to be stored subcutaneously in the buttocks, thighs, and hips. Men are more likely to have fat stored in the belly and lower back, due to sex hormone differences. When women reach menopause and the oestrogen produced by ovaries declines, fat migrates from their buttocks, hips and thighs to their waists. Later in life, fat is stored in the belly.

Fat Fact 4:

An excess of visceral fat (packed around organs) is known as central obesity, or "pregnant man syndrome", in which the abdomen protrudes excessively. There is a **strong** correlation between central obesity and cardiovascular disease.

Fat Fact 5:

Fat does not use much energy to be stored. Your body has to work very hard to convert carbohydrates into fat, whereas fat is already fat, and slides into adipose tissue with ease. In fact, your body can hardly resist storing dietary fat – it is a survival mechanism for times of famine.

Fat Fact 6:

As your body stores more fat, the number of fat cells remains the same, they just increase in size. This is because after puberty, you are stuck with the same number of fat cells in your body for the rest of your life. Unless you get liposuction (sucking out of fat cells) or become obese (the body is forced to make more fat cells).

This is the primary reason so many people who go on a diet, pack on the kilos straight afterwards. They think that they are getting rid of the fat cells, where in fact they are just emptying them. The fat cells remain there waiting to be refilled, which is why it is so important to maintain a *consistently* healthy lifestyle.

Fat Fact 7:

There are 4 different types of *dietary fat*.

- Saturated Fats (Bad Fats)

- Trans Fats (Very Bad Fats)

- Monounsaturated Fats (Good Fats)

- Polyunsaturated Fats (Good Fats)

Fat Fact 8:

In the next chapter, we will learn about the bad fats, and after that we will cover the good ones so that you become an expert in the field of fats, a very interesting subject, professor!

Degree Shift 18 –
Bad Fats (saturated)

There are 4 different types of *dietary fat*.

- Saturated Fats (Bad Fats)

- Trans Fats (Very Bad Fats)

- Monounsaturated Fats (Good Fats)

- Polyunsaturated Fats (Good Fats)

Saturated fats are often referred to as 'bad fats' because they are not considered essential for good health, and have been linked with an increased risk of heart disease and higher total cholesterol levels in the body.

Identifying saturated fats is quite easy, because they are solid at room temperature. Remember the last time you pulled some leftovers from the fridge and had to scrape a layer of fat off the top? You just caught some saturated fat trying to get into your arteries! They are mainly found in animal products but can be found in some plant sources.

Animal-based sources of saturated fats include:

- Dairy foods – such as butter, cream, milk and cheese

- Meat (such as fatty cuts of beef, pork and lamb, and processed meats like salami) and chicken (especially chicken skin)

Some plant-derived saturated fats include:

- Cooking margarine

- Coconut milk and coconut cream

Saturated fats are also commonly found in many manufactured and packaged foods such as:

- Fatty snack foods

- Deep fried take away foods

- Cakes

- Biscuits

- Pastries and pies

Saturated fats are one of the main causes of high blood cholesterol levels. The Heart Foundation has found that increasing amounts of saturated fats in your diet will cause a rise in the amount of 'bad cholesterol' in your blood and decrease the levels of 'good cholesterol'. This can cause sticky, fatty deposits to build up in your arteries, causing them to narrow - and this increases the risk of blockages. If this happens around the heart, it can cause a heart attack, and if it happens in the brain it can cause a stroke.

It is important to choose foods that are low in saturated fat to help ensure good health.

The Australian Government has made it mandatory for food manufacturers to list the amount of saturated fat in their products.

When choosing your foods, compare which product is better for you. Choose the product with the lowest saturated fat content in the per 100g column.

In the next chapter we will look at good fats. But in the mean time, remember that saturated fats are:

- Solid at room temperature

- Found in dairy, meat cuts and coconut

- Listed on all food labels

- Cause cholesterol to build up in your arteries and can cause heart attacks or strokes

Saturated fat killing tip: Chicken skin is very high in saturated fat. Pull all of the skin off a roast chicken before eating it, not while you eat it. If you pull it off while you eat it, you may find a little bit jumps out of your hand, into your mouth and down your throat!

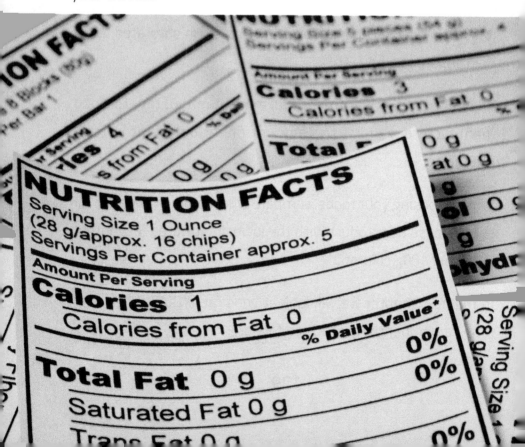

Degree Shift 19 – Good Fats (unsaturated)

There are 4 different types of *dietary fat*. In the last chapter, we looked at saturated fat. In this chapter we will look at the two *un*saturated fats.

Unsaturated fats are considered the 'healthy' fats and are encouraged as part of a healthy diet. These fats help reduce heart disease, lower cholesterol levels and have other health benefits **when they replace saturated fats in the diet**. This is important to understand. The TV adverts about special margarines improving your health can be misleading. They can improve your health if you substitute butter with margarine. If you don't have a butter addiction, don't add canola into your diet! If you already do have a butter addiction, is it really good if you substitute 'bad' with 'not so bad'? There are that many chemical additives in margarine that animals will not eat it – not even ants. There are much better ways to get your unsaturated fat.

You can tell the difference between saturated (bad) and unsaturated (good) fat, because good fats are liquid at room temperature, whereas bad fats are solid.

There are two types of unsaturated fats. Monounsaturated and polyunsaturated. These differ in their chemical structure and have slightly different health benefits as a result.

Sources of **monounsaturated** fats include:

- Olive oil

- Canola oil

- Peanut oil

- Nuts (such as cashews and almonds)

- Avocados

Replacing saturated fats with monounsaturated fats has a cholesterol lowering effect, but this is not to the same extent as polyunsaturated fats.

Polyunsaturated fats can be divided into two groups: Omega-3 and Omega-6. These two types of polyunsaturated fats have slightly different health benefits.

Omega-3 Fats

Omega-3 fats have been shown to be protective against heart disease and to help decrease bad cholesterol levels. Omega-3 fats are found in:

- Oily fish (such as salmon, sardines and blue-eye trevalla)

- Eggs and meats (such as lean beef and chicken)

- Plant sources (including linseed/flaxseed, walnuts, soybeans and canola oil).

Research has found that people who have a higher intake of fish have less risk of developing heart disease. Fish and other animal sources contain different types of Omega-3 fats to plant sources. The body is able to use the Omega-3 fats from animal sources better than from plant sources.

This means that to get the same benefits as you get from animal-based Omega-3 fats, you'd need to eat more plant-based Omega-3 fats. Omega-3's from animal sources have also been shown to have more benefits for cardiovascular health than plant Omega-3's.

Even though fish sources of Omega-3's have great benefits for heart health, pregnant and breastfeeding women must not consume more than the recommended amounts of fish due to the risk of consuming too much mercury from the fish.

The Heart Foundation recommends adults have 500mg of Omega-3 (marine source) everyday to reduce their risk of heart disease. For people who already have heart disease, The Heart Foundation recommends you have about 1,000mg of Omega-3 (marine source) everyday. To make it easier for you, you can now buy fish oil tablets, but remember that nothing is better than the real thing.

Omega-6 Fats

Omega-6 fats have been shown to decrease the risk of heart disease when they are consumed in place of saturated and trans fats. Omega-6 fat sources include:

- Sunflower, soybean, sesame oils

- Nuts (such as walnuts, pecans, brazil and pine nuts)

- Sunflower seeds.

Your task for this chapter is to ensure that you get 500mg of Omega-3 every day. Look at the food labels, and calculate your consumption. Please fill in the following table, explaining where you got your Omega-3 from.

Day:	Amount of Omega-3:	How I got it:
1		
2		
3		
4		
5		
6		
7		

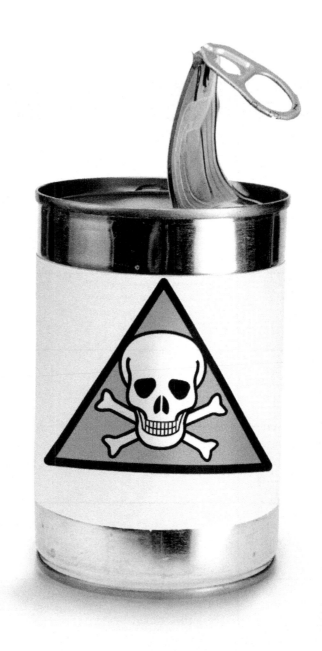

Degree Shift 20 – Pure Evil Fat

THERE are 4 different types of *dietary fat*. In the last chapter, we looked at unsaturated fats. In the previous chapter, we learned about saturated fats.

Just to recap:

- Saturated fats are BAD fats, and can be identified easily because they are solid at room temperature

- Unsaturated fats are GOOD fats, and are liquid at room temperature. There are two types; monounsaturated and polyunsaturated. Polyunsaturated fats are split into Omega 3 and 6 – which reduce the risk of heart diseases when replacing saturated fats in a diet.

This time, we are going to learn about the most disgusting of all fats. Trans fat.

Don't you just hate it when people lie to you? There is no reason for lying. Being told the truth is so much better in the long run, as it may cause short term pain, but compared to a lie, will not sever long term relationships – this is because relationships are built on trust.

One of the worst kind of lies is one where someone pretends to be someone that they are not. They put up a big show; put a lot of effort into being nice to you, when secretly they just want to hurt you. Don't you just hate people like that?

Trans fats are like those people. They are unsaturated fats that act like saturated fats in your body. They are good fats gone bad. They are the fats that went to private school and got A's in university, and are now knocking grannies over and stealing their handbags - all while pretending to be upstanding citizens of the food community.

Trans fats are unsaturated but, unlike the 'good' unsaturated fatty acids found in fish and vegetable oils, behave similarly to saturated fats in the body and have similar health issues.

Trans fats are created through an industrial process called hydrogenation. Hydrogenation is widely used to solidify liquid vegetable oils to make products such as margarines and shortenings and involves adding hydrogen to the oils at high temperature.

Trans fats are **uncommon in nature** but may be found in low levels in the fat of beef, lamb and dairy foods.

What makes trans fats so bad, other than their deceptive ways? Well, to understand, you need to know first that there are two types of cholesterol in your blood. Good and bad. (We will cover cholesterol in *Degree Shift 21*, but for the meantime, know that your goal is to increase good cholesterol, and reduce bad cholesterol)

We already know that unsaturated fats increase *good* cholesterol. We also know that saturated fats increase *bad* cholesterol. But what makes trans fats the godfather of all fats is that it increases bad cholesterol, while *at the same time* reduces good cholesterol!

The Heart Foundation has found that trans fats intake is associated with an increased risk of having heart attacks and heart disease. On January 1st 2010, California became the first place on earth to ban restaurants and bakeries from using cooking oils that contain trans fats.

Now if you don't already hate trans fats, read on:

Australian manufacturers are **not required** to include trans fats on food labels. It is mandatory to include total fat and saturated fat, but not trans fats!

It is important to be aware of the types of foods that may contain trans fats as it may not be obvious by looking at labels on food packages. Trans fats are found in deep fried fast foods and processed foods, like cakes and biscuits made with margarine and shortening.

If you do choose to eat foods such as margarine or foods that contain shortening, look for products that actually declare the trans fat content on the label, and choose the product with the lowest amount. If a product contains 'hydrogenated vegetable oil' or 'vegetable shortening' in the ingredients list; it contains trans fats.

Here are some useful tips on how to reduce your intake of trans fat:

- Avoid deep-fried fast foods and takeaways

- Limit manufactured biscuits, cakes and pies

- If you're eating margarine, choose those that are lowest in trans fatty acids

Your task this chapter is to be a food detective. Find those slimy trans fats, and banish them from your pantry or fridge. Write down where you discovered your trans fats hiding:

I found trans fats in:

And Like Arnold Schwarzenegger and the state of California, I declare a ban on trans fats in my diet!

Signed:

Name:

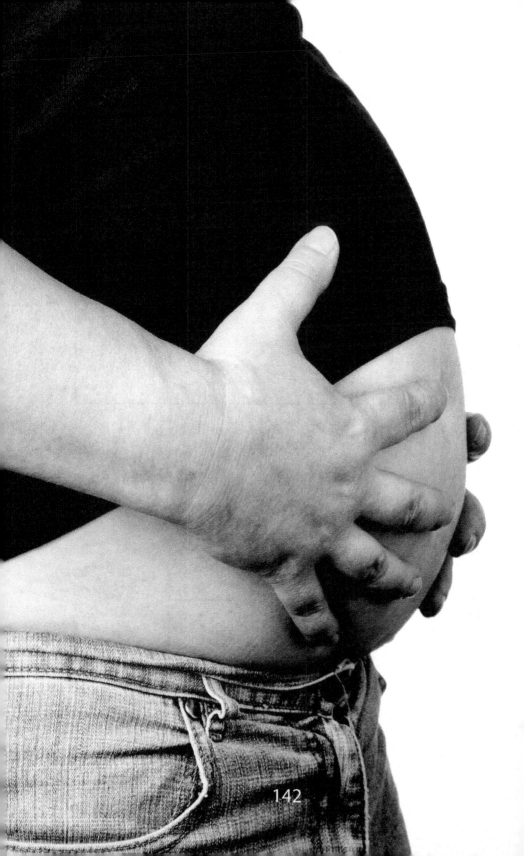

Degree Shift 21 - Cholesterol

CHOLESTEROL is a type of fat that is part of all animal cells. It is produced by the liver and also made by most cells in the body. Cholesterol may have been given a bad name in recent years, but you actually need blood cholesterol because it is essential to:

- Build the structure of cell membranes

- Make hormones like oestrogen, testosterone and adrenaline

- Help your metabolism work efficiently; for example, cholesterol is essential for your body to produce vitamin D

- Produce bile acids, which help the body digest fat and absorb important nutrients.

There are two types of cholesterol – good cholesterol and bad cholesterol.

- **Bad cholesterol** is called low density lipoprotein (LDL) cholesterol. LDL carries most of the cholesterol that is delivered to cells

- **Good cholesterol** is called high density lipoprotein (HDL), and helps remove excess cholesterol out of the cells, including cells in the arteries

Health authorities recommend that cholesterol levels should be no higher than 5.5mmols per litre, if there are no other risk factors present. The Heart Foundation says that approximately half of all adult Australians have a blood cholesterol level above 5.5mmols per litre, making high blood cholesterol a major health concern in Australia.

What makes cholesterol so bad? Well, as we have already learnt, when we eat saturated and trans fats, our bodies love to store them, giving them a 'free pass' to the blood stream so they can find a nice comfortable storage spot. But riding on the back of these fats are bad cholesterols.

Once in the blood stream, the bad cholesterol molecules, like unemployed troublemakers, hang around the walls of the arteries, getting in the way of the working blood cells as they rush about their important business. Too many of these troublemakers in one alleyway, could block the flow of workers and cause a disruption to the usual course of business. Unlike in the outside world, your blood needs to flow well, all the time. One blockage, for even a short time, could cause a major trauma, called a heart attack or stroke.

Good cholesterol is like a policeman; it clears out the bad cholesterol, one troublemaker at a time, and sends them off to prison, on big brown prison buses. Exercise is like the army in a time of war – it provides employment for bad cholesterol, forcing it to do the job it was created for, which then clears the arteries of their loitering.

Therefore exercise and healthy eating can reduce levels of bad cholesterol in your blood, so that your body can return to being a finely tuned machine. Unless you allow more in!

And if you are not convinced, please understand this: Your body can (and does) produce all the cholesterol it needs, you do not need to find cholesterol in your foods.

The Heart Foundation recommends the following to reduce your LDL (bad) cholesterol:

- Cease alcohol consumption or reduce your alcohol intake to no more than one or two drinks a day

- Don't smoke. Smoking increases the ability of LDL cholesterol to get into artery cells and cause damage

- Exercise regularly (for example, at least 30 minutes of brisk walking daily). Exercise increases the HDL levels, while reducing LDL levels in the body

- Lose any excess body fat. Being overweight may contribute to raised blood LDL levels

The Heart Foundation also states that total fat intake, especially saturated fat and trans fat, plays a larger role in blood cholesterol than intake of cholesterol itself. The Heart Foundation says that seafood contains some cholesterol, but is low in saturated fat and also contains healthy Omega-3 fatty acids. Fresh seafood (not fried or battered!) is a healthy food and should not be avoided just because it contains cholesterol.

For some people diet and lifestyle changes are not enough. High blood cholesterol levels often have a genetic component. Some people inherit altered genes that cause high cholesterol and require medication (as well as exercise and healthy eating) to reduce cholesterol.

Your task for this *Degree Shift* is to find out your blood cholesterol level. It is a very honest and revealing thing to find out, and just like a mole scan, should be something that you check regularly.

It may take a bit of time out of your day, but it is better than taking a lot of time off the end of your days. If you have already had a blood test for LDL levels, then go again – after a few weeks of healthy living, you will not only be looking better on the outside, but your doctor could show you how much better you are on the inside. Like winning an award for a competition you never thought you had even entered!

My cholesterol levels are:

P.S. In the next chapter we will review everything we have learnt about fats, so that we can move on with our journey, and learn about the building blocks of power – protein!

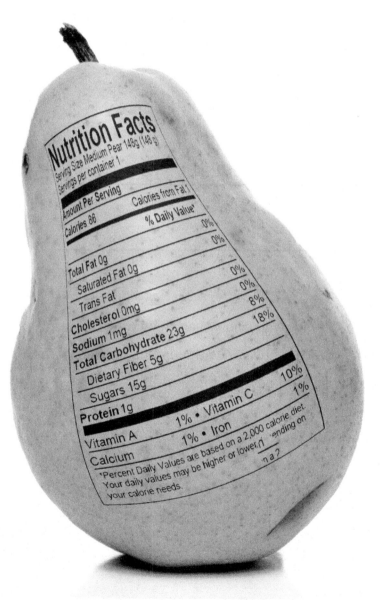

Nutrition Facts

Serving Size Medium Pear 148g (148 g)
Servings per container 1

Amount Per Serving

Calories from Fat 1

Calories 86

	% Daily Value*
	0%
	0%
Total Fat 0g	
Saturated Fat 0g	0%
Trans Fat	0%
Cholesterol 0mg	8%
Sodium 1mg	18%
Total Carbohydrate 23g	
Dietary Fiber 5g	
Sugars 15g	10%
Protein 1g	1%

Vitamin A   1% • Vitamin C

Calcium   1% • Iron

*Percent Daily Values are based on a 2,000 calorie diet.
Your daily values may be higher or lower, ...ending on
your calorie needs.

148

Degree Shift 22 –
Pressure

JOE Dispenza DC, author of the book "Evolve your mind" explains that the best way to learn something is to repeatedly fire the neuron pathways in the brain in the same way, so that they can 'remember' what you have learnt. We non brain surgeons call this practice. Nothing new here, we all know that you need to practice to master something. What you might *not* know, is that emotions are the anchor to your memories.

If you think back to being on a beach as a child, what do you remember? Above all else, you remember the emotions – happiness, joy, excitement. And how do you remember those emotions? Do you re-feel them?

We are going to use this theory right now, so that we can seal in the fat learnings, so that you will never forget them. Ever.

Using the most powerful of memory emotions – pressure.

Set an alarm to go off in 5 minutes. You are already running out of time. The following are 20 questions that you need to answer, otherwise you will be put back to *Never Diet Again 17*. You now have approximately 4 minutes. Go.

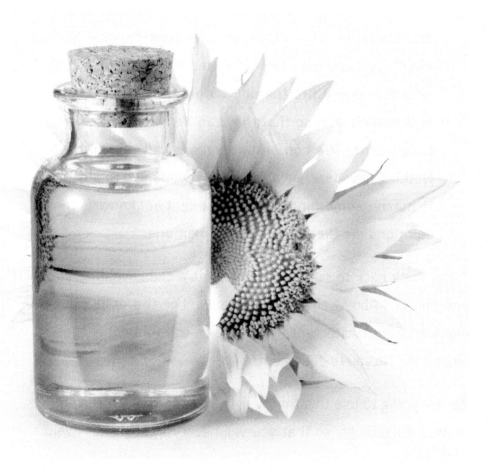

After puberty, the number of fat cells in the normal human body remains the same, they just change size.	True / false
It takes a lot of energy to store fat	True / false
A man with a big, rounded Homer Simpson belly is: A:) Sexy B:) Pregnant C:) At a high risk of heart disease	A / B / C
This is because: A:) He is healthy B:) He is yellow C:) He has fat packed tightly around his organs	A / B / C
Saturated fat is solid at room temperature	True / False

Rank these fats from best to worst (1 best, to 4 worst): Saturated Fat Trans Fat Monounsaturated Fat Polyunsaturated Fat	
Unsaturated fat is solid at room temperature	True / False
Saturated Fat is mostly found in: A:) Meat, dairy and coconut B:) Plants, nuts and fish	A / B
Unsaturated fat is found mostly in: A:) Meat, dairy and coconut B:) Plants, nuts and fish	A / B

Chicken skin is high in what type of fat? A:) Saturated Fat B:) Trans Fat C:) Monounsaturated D:) Polyunsaturated	A / B / C / D
The Australian Government has made it mandatory to list Saturated Fat content on food labels	True / False
The Australian Government has made it mandatory to list Trans Fat content on food labels	True / False

The Heart Foundation recommends adults have ___**mg of Omega-3 (marine source) every day.** A:) 0 B:) 1 C:) 500 D:) 10,000	A / B / C / D
TV ads tell you to eat special cholesterol reducing margarine. Holistically speaking, what is the healthiest option below: A:) Start adding margarine to your diet B:) Start eating margarine instead of butter C:) Don't eat margarine or butter	A / B / C
Trans fats are common in nature	True / False
Trans fats are so bad that they scare *Terminator* **and** *Robocop*	True / False

Because trans fat levels do not have to be listed in the food label, I should look for what in the ingredients list? A:) Hydrogenated vegetable oil B:) Shortening C:) Partially hydrogenated vegetable oil D:) Vegetable shortening E:) All of the above	A / B / C / D / E
Approximately half of Australian adults have blood cholesterol higher than 5.5mmols per litre, making high blood cholesterol a major health concern	True / False
Bad cholesterol is like an unemployed troublemaker, good cholesterol is like a policeman, and exercise is like the army.	True / False

To live a healthier, longer life I have committed to reducing saturated fats, banning trans fats, eating 500mg of Omega-3 per day, exercising regularly and losing (and keeping off) any excess body fat.	True / False
I will always remember my fat facts, so that I can eliminate ignorance as an excuse for an unhealthy life	True / False

Now that you have completed your test, you need to understand that you would not have been put down to *Degree Shift 17*; the point was to put you under pressure, so that you would associate "high pressure" as an emotional anchor to fat. The reason that pressure is the most powerful of memory emotions is that it also forces you to focus on the task at hand.

Now, when you think of cakes, pies, chicken skin or any other bad fat, you will subconsciously feel high pressure, instead of hunger. And you won't even be able to help it!

One more automatic weapon in your health holster.

Degree Shift 23 -
Protein

CONGRATULATIONS on doing so well on your exam! Would you have thought a few weeks ago that you could have answered 20 questions about fat without warning? This time we will learn about the building blocks of the human body - protein.

The best sources of protein are beef, poultry, fish, eggs, dairy products, nuts, seeds, and legumes like black beans and lentils. Protein's job is to build, maintain, and replace the tissues in your body. As a fitness junkie, you might think that protein is only good for building muscle, but it does so much more than that! Your organs, your blood and your immune system are made up of protein.

To describe proteins as accurately as possible – imagine you zoomed right in on a food protein source (for example a beef steak). You would see that it was made up of a whole bunch of Lego pieces, like an intricate Lego toy – a pirate ship for example. If you eat that piece of steak, your digestive system breaks the pirate ship into its individual pieces of Lego, which then pass into the blood stream, where the ship can be rebuilt.

What is exciting, however – is that your body is like a Lego genius – and has the plans for any kind of Lego creation it might feel like building. All it needs is the pieces, and it can do the rest. Like Lego, there are literally thousands of different pieces to build from – but 22 of them are used the most. These building blocks are called amino acids – and of the 22 important amino acids, the body actually manufactures 13 of them – leaving you to find the other 9 from your diet.

Side note: Have you ever heard the term *essential* in foods – such as *essential amino acids* or *essential vitamins*? If something is essential, it means that the body cannot make it by itself – it needs to find it from food. *So the 9 missing amino acids are called the essential amino acids.*

Protein from an animal source, such as meat or milk, is called complete, because it contains all nine of the essential amino acids. Most vegetable protein is considered incomplete because it lacks one or more of the essential amino acids. This can be a concern for someone who doesn't eat meat or milk products.

People who eat a vegetarian diet can still get all their essential amino acids by eating a wide variety of protein-rich vegetable foods. For instance, you can't get all the amino acids you need from peanuts alone, but if you have peanut butter on whole-grain bread you're covered. Likewise, red beans won't give you everything you need, but red beans and rice can do the trick. The good news is that you don't have to eat all the essential amino acids in every meal. As long as you have a variety of protein sources throughout the day, your body will grab what it needs from each meal.

According to the National Health and Medical Research Council of Australia (the people who say what %RDI figures are on food labels), the average adult needs 1g of complete protein per kg of body weight in their diet every day. So if you weigh 70kg, you need 70g of protein. This week, your job is to track how much protein you eat.

Day	Protein	Sources	Notes and observations

Degree Shift 24 – Amino Acids

IN chapter 23, we mentioned essential amino acids. Remember, there are 9 of them, and they are called essential because the body needs them, but cannot manufacture them – so we need to get them from our food.

You may have wondered what these 9 amino acids are, where they come from, and what they are used for – so let's uncover the secrets of these fancy little things. Put on your lab coat, strap on some safety goggles, we're going to tick them off one by one, and see how important they really are...

Phenylalanine serves in the body as a precursor to the catecholamine family of hormones. What this technical mumbo jumbo means is that the hormone adrenalin (and its sister noradrenalin) is made from phenylalanine. Food sources or phenylalanine are dairy, almonds, avocados, lima beans, peanuts, and seeds. Interestingly, most artificial sweeteners contain phenylalanine, which taken in large doses causes "weepy bum" as it loosens your sphincter. Maybe better to have your coffee plain?

Threonine is important for antibody production. Antibodies are the detectives in your body – cruising your bloodstream looking for threats, such as viruses and bacteria. Threonine can also be converted into glycine – a non-essential amino acid which is responsible for building your DNA correctly, as well as preventing muscle breakdown. Quite important? We absolutely think so! Dietary sources of threonine include dairy, beef, poultry, eggs, beans, nuts, and seeds.

Valine is needed for muscle metabolism, tissue repair, and for the maintenance of proper nitrogen balance in the body. Valine is found in high concentrations in the muscle tissue. It is also one of the three branched chain amino acids (BCAA's), which means that it can be used as an energy source by muscle tissue. Valine may also be helpful in treating liver and gallbladder disorders. Dietary sources of valine include dairy products, grain, meat, mushrooms, peanuts, and soy proteins.

Leucine stimulates muscle protein synthesis (building muscle) and, being the second of our BCAA's is also used as a fuel – primarily in anabolic (growth) reactions. So this is the BCAA that is hard at work the night after a strength training session. Interestingly, during times of starvation, stress, infection, or recovery from trauma, the body uses leucine to aid in the healing process. Insulin deficiency is known to result in poor utilisation of leucine; therefore, diabetics may require higher levels of leucine intake. Leucine is found in cottage cheese, sesame seeds, peanuts, dry lentils, chicken, and fish.

Isoleucine is our third BCAA, and is important for blood sugar regulation, muscle development and repair, haemoglobin development, and energy regulation. To understand how important isoleucine is, we need to look at what happens when we don't have enough. A deficiency in isoleucine results in dizziness, headaches, fatigue, depression, confusion and irritability. Next time you feel like this, you may have not eaten enough isoleucine, which is found in eggs, fish, lentils, poultry, beef, seeds, soy, wheat, almonds and dairy.

Tryptophan is one of the building blocks of serotonin and melatonin. It is plentiful in chocolate, oats, bananas, dried dates, milk, cottage cheese, meat, fish, turkey and peanuts.

Serotonin has two jobs – one is to transmit messages from nerve to nerve, and the other is to cause blood vessels to shut when they have been cut (so that we don't bleed to death). Serotonin intake can actually alter your mood – it is prescribed for patients with depression, and is the main reason that people love chocolate.

Melatonin is responsible for adequate sleep, as well as regulation of a diverse number of body functions. It is released prior to bed (as it gets dark) and suppressed as it gets lighter. It has been suggested that night shift workers have shorter life spans because they do not have regular melatonin release.

Chemically speaking, when we have insulin in the blood (after a high GI carb hit), all amino acids in the blood get shunted into cells – except tryptophan, which stays in the blood and is in a relatively higher concentration (because there is nothing else there) – this is why kids feel so happy when they eat sugary foods.

Lysine is one of the building blocks of niacin (Vitamin B). Low levels of niacin can cause the disease pellagra. Pellagra is a serious, disgusting and deadly disease found mostly in countries whose staple diet is corn. This is why it is advertised as added to corn flakes, as corn is a low source of lysine (and tryptophan!). It is also the main medication used in the treatment and prevention of herpes (cold sores). Lysine sources include green beans, lentils, soybean, and spinach.

Methionine supplies sulphur and other compounds required by the body for normal metabolism and growth. It belongs to a group of compounds, called lipotropics, which help the liver process fats. It is found in fish, whole grains, and dairy.

Glutamine is technically not an essential amino acid, because it can be manufactured by the body, it is however the most abundantly occurring amino acid, and is considered conditionally essential because we may not be able to manufacture enough when building muscle. Glutamine is found circulating in your blood and in your muscles, and is known as the healer in the body. A high intake of glutamine after surgery or illness speeds up recovery dramatically.

So, do you now understand how important it is to have an adequate intake of protein? This brings a new meaning to the term "essential"!

In the next chapter, we will look into protein shakes.

Degree Shift 25 – What's in my protein shake?

As you might imagine, after a strength training session, you have put your body under stress, and it needs the building blocks (amino acids) found in proteins to rebuild the muscles that have been worked. Your body needs to rebuild them to be stronger, so that the same amount of stress (weight) will not cause the same amount of damage next time you have to lift it.

So far, we have looked at a few natural sources of protein – for example a grilled rump steak (fat cut off) has about 28% protein. As we discussed in *Degree Shift 23*, a 70kg person needs 70g of complete protein in their diet every day. If we do the maths, this would mean that the 70kg person would need 250g of steak per day. Now take into consideration that lean steak has a fat content of around 6%, so to get your 70g of protein, you would have to eat 15g of fat. This is very interesting, especially knowing that animal fat is mostly saturated fat (so very easily stored, and contains bad cholesterol).

If we then have a bit of fun and project out a bit further, 15g of fat per day for a whole year equates to nearly 5kg of pure saturated fat. Walk with us a little while as we play further with the mathematics. 5kg of fat contains 49,275 calories. To burn off this many calories, you would need to walk briskly for close to 200 hours. That is 30 minutes of brisk walking every single day just to use up the fat that you had to ingest to get the protein that you needed.

It gets even more interesting when you realise that brisk walking doesn't just burn the fat. Brisk walking burns 50% fat and 50% carbohydrates (remember that carbohydrates are stored as glycogen). So one hour of daily walking before you are actually reducing your body fat! **Side note** – running burns 30% fat and 70% glycogen.

Can you see now how there would be a market for a low fat protein source? How about a product that was a higher percentage protein by weight – so that a 70kg person would just have to eat 70g of steak to get 70g of protein? It would be nice to then use that hour of walking to reduce our body fat percentage, rather than to just stall it. And if we were at our perfect body fat level, wouldn't it be nice to use that walking to burn off something that we actually wanted to eat?

Thankfully there is such a product, and yes – it is in your protein shake. But we wouldn't cheat you out of some knowledge by just stopping there! Let's find out what a protein shake really is...

Put simply, protein shakes are created as a by-product of cheese manufacture. Did you know that cheese is made from letting milk go sour? What happens is that the milk forms lumps (called curds). The watery, grey liquid that the curds float in is called whey. Remember Little Miss Muffet? Curds and whey is in fact cottage cheese – curds that have not been completely drained of the whey.

Whey contains lactose, traces of fat, minerals, vitamins and a high percentage of complete protein in a water suspension.

(Imagine how much protein a calf would need to get from milk in order to grow as fast as it does?)

This whey is not poured into a cup and given to you, however. It is first microfiltered (to get rid of the fat) and dried (to get rid of the water) leaving a powder called whey protein concentrate. Whey protein concentrate (WPC) contains between 29% and 89% protein by weight. This variation is because it still contains carbohydrates (in the form of lactose). So, we have a product that has around the same (or more) protein than a lean steak, but a lot less fat.

Let's take it a step further.

Whey Protein Isolate (WPI) is a purer form of protein made by isolating the protein molecules in WPC (by removing the lactose and fat). WPI is more than 90% protein, and is therefore digested much quicker than WPC.

WPI and WPC can be bought in powder form, and taste milky when mixed with water. Many companies add flavour to "whey" in order to make it easier to drink. WPI requires more labour to produce, and is therefore more expensive than WPC. Unfortunately the isolation process reduces the bioavailability of some of the amino acids that make up the protein. If it weren't for this, you would obviously pay the extra to get the purer WPI.

If we take the production of whey further, we can create a substance called hydrolysed whey protein. This is done by partially digesting the protein using chemicals, in turn making the protein able to be digested in the human body nearly instantly. The drawback of this is that hydrolysed whey protein tastes very, very bitter and is much more expensive, so generally not seen on the shelves.

There is another form of protein that can be made from milk, called casein. Casein is actually made from curds, by removing the fat and then drying them to a powdered form. Casein has traditionally been used as a glue in cabinet making, and as you can imagine becomes a gluey sticky substance in your gut when you eat it. So while WPI and WPC are fast absorbing, Casein is the protein equivalent of complex carbohydrate. It takes up to 7 hours to digest. Casein also has a higher bioavailability of amino acids than both WPI and WPC.

So, WPI would be best consumed straight after strenuous exercise to get into the muscles as fast as possible. (Hydrolysed, whey would be faster but too hard to keep down) WPC would also need to be consumed to provide the missing amino acids due to their reduced bioavailability in WPI. Casein would also be good to have before bed, because the real muscle building occurs while we sleep.

Buying all of these can get quite expensive, so manufacturers have created the ultimate blend of the three proteins, combined with your favourite flavour to give you the protein that you need without giving you the fat that you don't want.

Leaves a nice taste in your mouth, doesn't it?

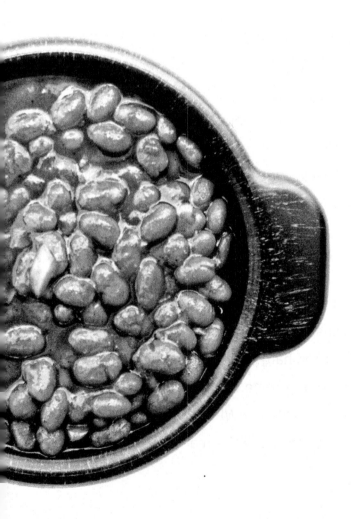

Degree Shift 26 - Fibre

"Beans, beans the musical fruit

The more you eat, the more you toot

The more you toot the happier you feel

So let's eat beans with every meal."

Do you remember that all carbohydrates are made up of glucose molecules bound together? The more molecules, and the more complex the structure, the harder the digestive system has to work to break it up into individual glucose molecules?

Sometimes, the structure of the carbohydrate is so complex that the body simply cannot digest it – no matter how long it spends crushing it in the stomach, or pumping it full of acid. It cannot break it down into glucose molecules, meaning that it passes unchanged from the stomach, through the small intestines, into the large intestine. A carbohydrate that is this complex is referred to as fibre.

We know now that our bodies are pretty resourceful, so we could ask two questions:

- Does it have another way of digesting this fibre?

- Or is there a good reason that we cannot digest this fibre?

To answer these questions, we first need to examine the types of fibre. Fibre is classified as either soluble (able to mix with water) or insoluble (does not hold water). The important thing to note before we categorise, is that most fibre sources contain both soluble and insoluble fibre. The message that you should take from today is that total fibre intake is what is important, no matter the type. There is however, a marked difference in the way each type of fibre is digested and therefore, how it affects us.

In the same way that a sponge does not mix with water (it is insoluble), insoluble fibre cannot mix with water, instead absorbing water to soften its passage through the bowels. Because of this, insoluble fibre is very filling (imagine eating a squashed up dry bath sponge, and how it would expand with the water in your stomach). Besides the reduction in calories from feeling full, this expansion makes it easier for the body to push food through the intestines. Imagine that the sponge that you ate is scraping the walls of your intestines, taking with it other food particles from previous meals – bringing meaning to the saying "cleaning you out".

Where insoluble fibre is the rough cleaner, soluble fibre is a bit more delicate, and performs some pretty amazing feats.

Soluble fibre, because it mixes with water to make a paste, actually slows down stomach emptying – making you feel fuller for longer, which ensures that sugar is released and absorbed more slowly. This means that soluble fibre effectively lowers the overall Glycaemic Index (GI) of carbohydrates.

Once mixed with water, soluble fibre attracts and binds to bile acids. Bile acids are a type of digestive acid that separates fats from food and transports them to the blood stream. By binding to soluble fibre, bile acids are rendered useless, meaning that the fat ends up "just passing through."

Pretty handy? What if I told you that your body manufactures bile acid from bad cholesterol? Therefore, by binding with soluble fibre, bile acid is lost. The body then replaces it by converting, and therefore using up, some of the cholesterol floating in our blood. This is how soluble fibre reduces LDL (bad) cholesterol.

Fibre is therefore quadrupley beneficial to your diet:

- It creates bulk in food, speeding up passage through the bowels

- It makes us feel fuller for longer, reducing GI of foods

- It reduces absorption of fat

- It lowers LDL cholesterol levels

The only downside is that fibre makes you fart. This is because dietary fibre moves largely unchanged into the large intestine or colon where it is fermented by friendly bacteria that live there. The fermentation process creates a gas with a sometimes potent smell.

Most people who begin to eat the correct amount of fibre are embarrassed by the farting. The smell is worse initially because the first bit of fibre acts like a drain cleaner, pushing a lot of old food particles into the large intestine, really adding to the overall potence of your proud fart. If you are eating the correct amount of fibre regularly, the potence of the smell will go away after the first few days. Once this has happened, you have rid your body of some potentially toxic waste. "Better out than in," as grandad says!

This week, your job is to ensure that you eat the correct amount of fibre every day, and suffer the stench for a few days to potentially increase your life by a few years. It is recommended that Australians eat at least 30g of fibre per day – so add it up!

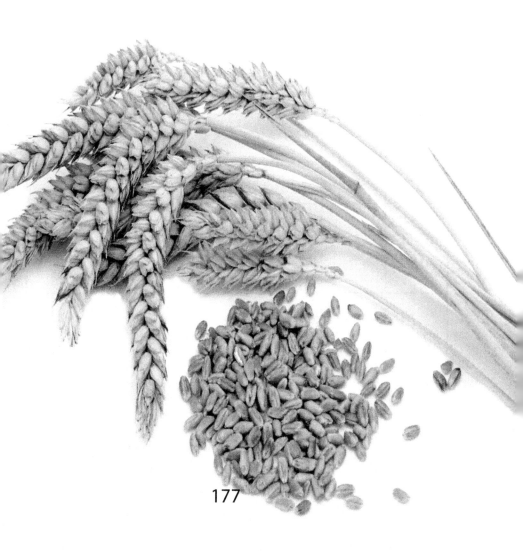

Day	Fibre	Sources	Notes and observations

Degree Shift 27 - Alcohol

WE now know that under normal conditions, your body gets its energy from the calories in carbohydrates, fats and proteins. We also know that to release these calories, the food needs to be digested, which uses energy. Even dextrose, the simplest digestible carbohydrate, needs some digestion.

Alcohol, on the other hand requires no digestion. It simply slips straight through the stomach to the small intestine, where it jumps the queue ahead of your normal food, straight to the blood stream. Once in the blood stream, your liver works very hard to rid your system of this poison, which means that there is no attention paid to the other foods in the blood. These carbohydrates and fats are therefore stored for later – as body fat.

All of this work affects the liver in some horrible ways. Being the biggest internal organ, it is readily known that it plays a key role in the major functions of the human body. Cirrhosis of the liver occurs when good, healthy organ tissue is replaced with bad scar tissue, due to constant overexposure to alcohol. This bad tissue then keeps the liver from having blood flow through, which in turn stops it from working properly.

While this is going on, the function of your kidneys has been distracted. Your kidneys are a blood filter – they catch all the nasty stuff in your blood (which is suspended in water). All the nasties are passed out as urine, and the water is put back into the blood stream on the other side. When alcohol is in the blood, your kidneys just pass everything out as urine – nasties, alcohol and water. This is why a hangover feels like dehydration – it is dehydration. After *Degree Shift 5* and *6*, you have personally experienced the importance of correct hydration to so many bodily functions.

If that's not bad enough, alcohol consumption prior to sleep reduces the quality of your sleep. Not only do you have to get up to urinate, but your body will only allow you deep, reparative sleep once the alcohol has been fully metabolised – one hour per standard drink. This means that if you were to have 6 beers before bed, you would not begin your deep sleep for 6 hours, which means in the morning, you feel as though you have only had 2 hours of sleep.

There are numerous other reasons to quit alcohol. Like how much of a fool you act when you drink, or how you say things you regret, or that dancing style that embarrasses your kids. Yes. That's right; we are going to ask you to quit drinking alcohol. For a whole year.

We have left this step to this late in the piece because many people put so much importance on their drinking. They have so many reasons as to why they drink. But remember it was only a couple of decades ago that people thought that smoking was cool, and even good for your health.

Your task is to tell at least 5 people that you no longer drink. Explain to them why alcohol is dangerous to your health. Explain to them that you no longer want hangovers. Explain that you want to enjoy the best part of the day (sunrise) whilst feeling the stronger euphoria of exercise. Explain to them that you care about your health, and want them to be supportive of your decision, and that you will be supportive if they choose to stop drinking as well. Ask them why they think that it is a good idea that you stop drinking. Record what they said on the next page:

Obviously, if you already do not drink then this step is completely irrelevant and you deserve to be congratulated. To some people, giving up social drinking is harder than anything they have ever endured in their lives.

Name:	What they said:

This is a very, very important step in your *Never Diet Again* journey. Even if you think it crazy and completely impossible to stop drinking for a whole year, just complete the exercise with conviction. The important thing is that the people you tell need to believe you.

If you do this exercise properly, a lot will be revealed as you tell your friends, and especially in the next chapter.

Interesting fact: the calories contained in one can of beer will take 42 minutes to walk off. That means to burn off a 6 pack of beer would take 4 hours and 15 minutes of walking – if that's all you had. Or, you could just run a half marathon.

How important is that drink to you?

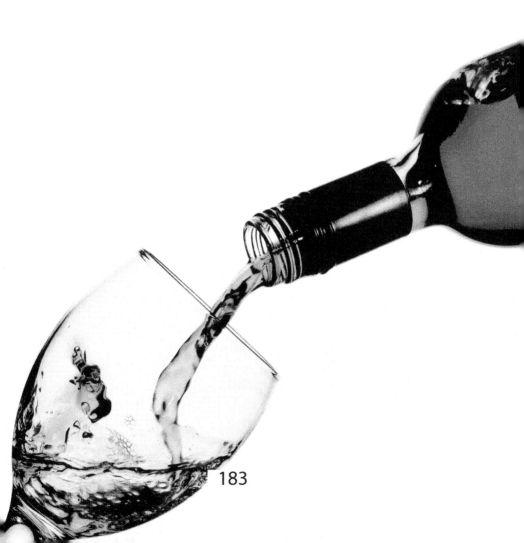

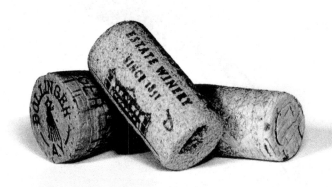

Degree Shift 28 – The French Paradox

WHAT is interesting about telling people that you no longer drink is how they respond. Check this out:

- If the person you told got defensive, changed the topic from you to them, seemed a bit panicky and gave you a lot of reasons why they could / would / should not stop drinking, then your friend is trying very hard to tell themselves that drinking is not a problem. Not very helpful to you though?

- If your friend told you that there is no way that you can cope, it is impossible for you to stay dry for a whole year, then your friend thinks you have a drinking problem.

- If your friends are supportive and keen to see you succeed, you have obviously given them reason to believe in you. Well done.

- If your friends think it is a great idea, and want to do it with you, then they not only believe in you, but find you inspirational.

- If your friends said "you don't even drink" then you did the exercise, even though you didn't have to. You are truly committed.

If you motivate an idiot, they just do stupid things faster.

Remember that *Never Diet Again* is education, not motivation. The motivation comes from within you. Nobody can give it to you, and nobody can take that away from you. We try to expose your inner inspiration, and provide you with education to allow your motivation to move you forward.

One of the most common justifications for why people drink is an offbeat reference to the "French Paradox". The French Paradox is a medical puzzle. Why is it that French people eat a high saturated fat diet, but have lower risk of heart disease than the US? It is an interesting question, so let's look into it.

The French Paradox was introduced to the world in 1991 on an episode of 60 minutes, where researches said that "the most probable cause of difference is that French drink red wine". Interestingly, red wine sales jumped 44%, and red wine companies began subtly getting the word out that red wine reduces the risk of heart disease. The theory being that red wine contains a chemical called resveratrol (a powerful antioxidant that comes from the skin of red grapes).

So immediately, we can eliminate beer drinking as a way to reduce heart disease, and for that matter white wine or spirits.

Since 1991, there has been a lot of publicity for this wonderfully convenient excuse to drink. Two very interesting books (*French Women Don't Get Fat* by Mireille Guiliano and *The Fat Fallacy* by Dr. Will Clower) both agree, however that red wine cannot be the only reason for the French Paradox. Their findings point to two very interesting observations.

- The French (unlike Australians and Americans) eat smaller portions, preferring quality to quantity. They put a lot of emphasis on the pleasure of taste, not on the pleasure of being full. Put simply, they just eat less.

- American and Australian diets are high in trans fat and sugar. Think about the high trans fat burger and fries, combined with the sugar (and resulting insulin spike) from the fizzy drink in most fast food joints. Sumo food?

The problem then, is that Americans heard this small snippet of information, subsequently increasing their alcohol consumption, resulting in the common misconception of "one drink per day keeps the heart attack away".

Consider this. Should you eat a healthy diet, with small regular portions which are low in bad fat and sugar, and combine this with regular exercise, why not have a glass of red wine every once in a while? Before you can answer this question, you need to ask yourself two far more important questions:

- Do you actually like the taste of wine?

- Can you have only one standard glass (100ml) at a time?

If you don't like the taste of wine, then why drink it? If you can't stop after 100ml (not much is it?), then you have an addiction. Harsh, but fair.

Herein lies the reason we asked you to stop drinking for a whole year. If you drink more than 100ml, or if you drink for the feeling of drunkenness, then you are drinking irresponsibly. You therefore need to learn to live without alcohol, so that in a year when you do start drinking again, you are used to not drinking, and can control yourself – drinking responsibly.

We both feel very strongly about alcohol abuse, and believe that the greatest problem is that it does not only affect your health. Drinking affects your relationships. By getting this far through *Never Diet Again*, you have become an inspiration to those around you, and you now have a responsibility to them. Find something that is satisfying to do for entertainment. After all, if drinking was good for you, why do hangovers hurt?

This is the last you will hear about alcohol from us. What you do with what we have given to you is your decision, and we will respect that. In the next chapter we will talk about antioxidants. What are they?

In the meantime, ponder the following: If I cannot even entertain the idea of giving up alcohol for a year, am I in control of alcohol, or does alcohol control me?

Be inspirational!

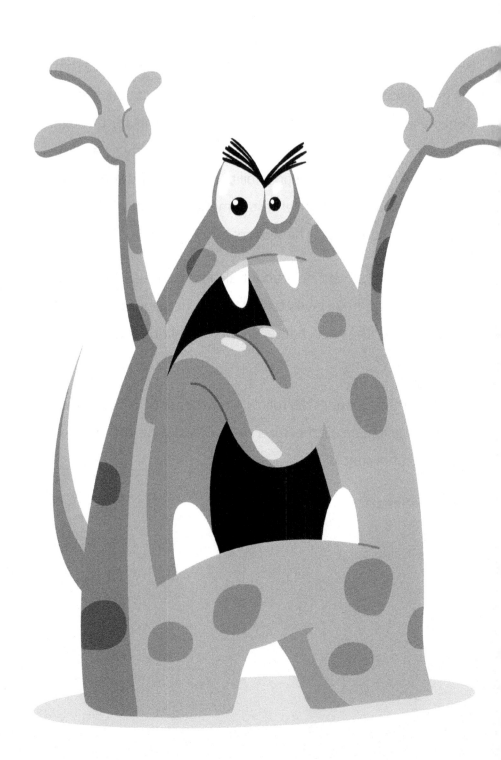

Degree Shift 29 - Antioxidants

WELL we know that antioxidants are important, and many 'health food' companies promote the antioxidant properties of their products. So let's find out what all the fuss is about...

Imagine that you live in the centre of a large city and last night, just up the road, a space ship crash landed, spilling hundreds of aliens into the city. These aliens are confused from the accident, cannot speak our language, and just roam around aimlessly, but angry. Imagine also, that these aliens are extremely volatile – exploding if they touch any solid object. If they walk into a wall, they explode, bringing down the building. Sometimes they hit a wall, and the resultant explosion starts a fire, which burns down an entire block.

Crazy as it may seem, this scenario is happening in your body right now. These aliens are called 'free radicals.' Free radicals cruise your body until they come into contact with a solid object (usually a cell wall). When they do, they explode, damaging the cell. Sometimes this explosion sets off a chain reaction, which destroys many surrounding cells – starting something rather sinister, that we call cancer.

As the mayor of your town, what do you do? You could wait for the aliens to all run into the buildings and blow up, leaving you with a lot of cleaning up to do, and many lives lost. You could wait for the army to arrive, but the result would be a war, which would use precious resources and potentially destroy the fabric of your fine city for years to come...

While you are pondering a solution to the problem, you notice that the aliens are extremely attracted to very bright colours. Red, yellow, green and orange being their absolute favourites. Being a fast decision maker, you decide it would be best to sacrifice all the city's bright coloured cars – by driving them into the vacant block, luring the aliens away from the buildings. The aliens begin to slowly destroy themselves, and all you had to do was sacrifice a few brightly coloured cars. You are lauded as a hero for making a small sacrifice for a greater cause. Well done!

Lucky for you, your brain is the mayor of the city that is your body. Only the cars are called antioxidants, and you replenish your stock of them by eating colourful fruits and vegetables. This is where 'a rainbow of colour' with your vegetables and fruits comes from. It's not just for fun, it's to survive! All you have to do is sacrifice a few colourful fruits and vegetables, and you can be lauded as the saviour of your own body!

Now for the interesting bit – how are free radicals created? How do these aliens get into my body?

Free radicals are created from external stimuli such as smoking, exposure to UV light, alcohol and pollution. Mmm, sinister. If I avoid the sun, smoking and pollution I'll avoid free radicals? Not quite. Free radicals are unfortunately also created from normal day to day processes. Breathing, aerobic exercise, metabolism, inflammation, emotions... the list goes on.

For all the chemistry geniuses – your body is kept alive by millions of chemical reactions. Sometimes, these reactions do not go full cycle, leaving a highly charged oxygen atom floating around.

Oxygen, in its elemental forms is a natural paradox. While oxygen is essential to support life – it is the "O" in the air (O_2) as well as in the water we drink (H_2O) – it is a highly unstable element, which reacts chemically with nearly anything. A good example of this is rust, also known as oxidation.

So if the alien metaphor is not good enough for you, just remember that a 'rainbow of colour' prevents internal rusting.

And what do most kids call something that is rusty?

Old.

This week, try to get a wide variety of colours in your fruit and vegetables every day.

Day	What colours I ate:
1	
2	
3	
4	
5	
6	
7	

Remember that fruit and vegetables provide your body with carbohydrate and fibre. Knowing now that they also possess antioxidant properties, you may be beginning to see why they are so important to your nutrition.

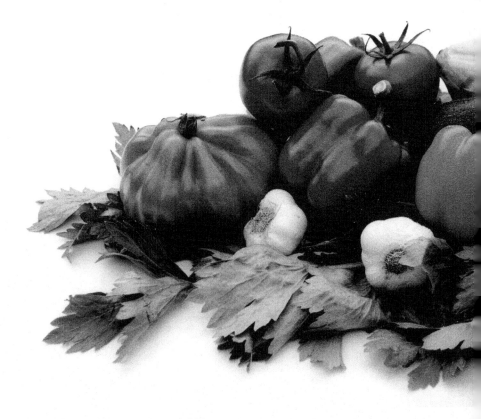

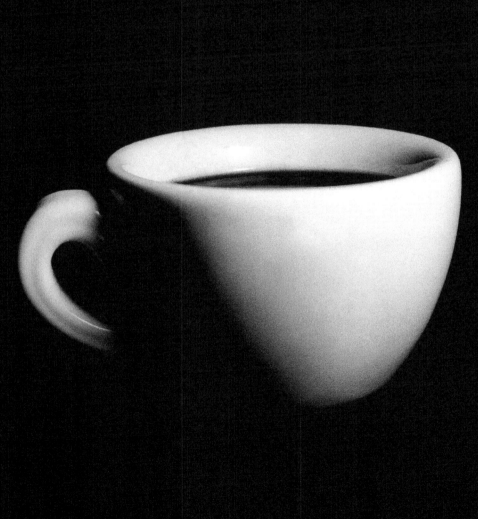

Degree Shift 30 – Coffee and Tea

"What a curse is it that ordinary working men should sit the whole day in coffee houses simply to chatter about politics, while their unhappy children are wailing at home for lack of bread?"

This was a petition more than 350 years ago, just before the British government began to tax coffee.

About 240 years ago, as a protest against oppression and excessive taxes, citizens of Boston boarded British ships moored in their harbour and tipped all their cargo overboard.

What was their cargo? Tea.

Since then, the United States has become the largest per capita coffee consuming nation on earth. And who is little brother to the USA?

Aussie! We have done everything to keep our big brother happy. Trade agreements since then have locked Australia as a major trading partner to the US. Now that America's economy is failing, Australia may look for a new mentor, or stand on its own two feet. Who knows?

"But I love coffee."

Alright, pull back a little, this chapter is about caffeine. Not coffee. What are the facts, so we can make up our own minds...?

Here are 4 things you need to know about caffeine:

- Caffeine as we all know so well does not eliminate the need for sleep; it only temporarily reduces the sensation of being tired.

- Studies have proven that caffeine increases physical output by 7 to 51% in trained athletes, so giving caffeine to a 10km runner will make them run for a further 5km at their race pace.

- Caffeine increases short term concentration, but reduces creative thought, and impairs long term memory. That's why you can't remember anything from university exams!

- Humans build a tolerance to caffeine within 7 days.

So to use caffeine more effectively, we should avoid it until we really need it. This could be the night before a deadline, or half an hour before an important sporting event. If we do this, we will have a low tolerance, and be able to use it to give ourselves that much needed kick. But like all drugs, caffeine is addictive...

Tea has all the benefits of coffee, as it contains caffeine, just in smaller doses. Tea also contains theanine, which in combination with caffeine has been known to stimulate alpha brain waves, calm the body and promote relaxed awareness. Tea allows your mind to be alert, yet rested – rather than the jittery sleeplessness of coffee. A cup of tea contains half the amount of caffeine that a standard cup of coffee contains.

Let's take it a step further. Green tea, made from undried tea leaves (rather than fully dried and processed tea leaves in traditional tea), contains very high concentrations of antioxidants, not found in coffee or tea.

We know the benefits of antioxidants, but here are two more things that you need to know about green tea.

- Catechins, found in green tea increase exercise endurance by allowing your body to burn fat whilst reducing glycogen utilisation.

- Green tea contains EGCG, which when combined with caffeine and theanine stimulates metabolism much more than coffee, because EGCG and caffeine work better together than they do individually.

So there you have it, if you want to be healthier, lose fat and exercise longer; drink green tea. If you need a pick me up, drink coffee. Green tea for long term wants, coffee for short term needs.

So we are not asking you to give up caffeine, you little druggy. Simply replace your regular coffee consumption with good quality green tea, and save the coffee for emergencies. Try it for a month and decide for yourself.

Final spanner: Coffee is a diuretic, meaning that it makes you urinate (dehydrate), whereas green tea is not, green tea consumption can count towards your daily water...

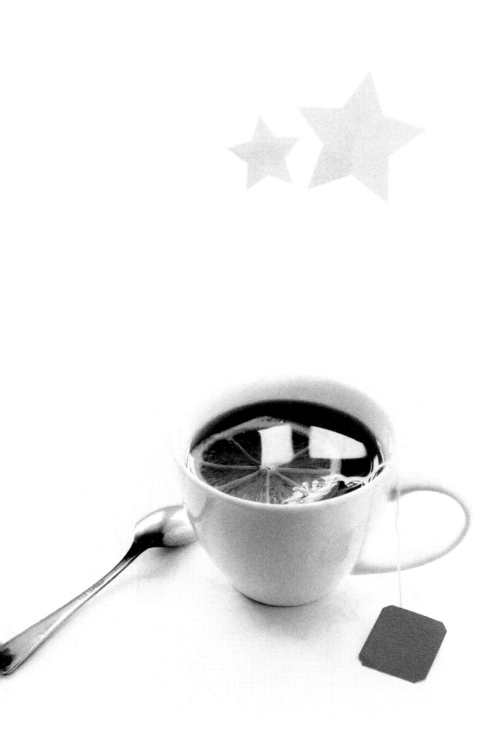

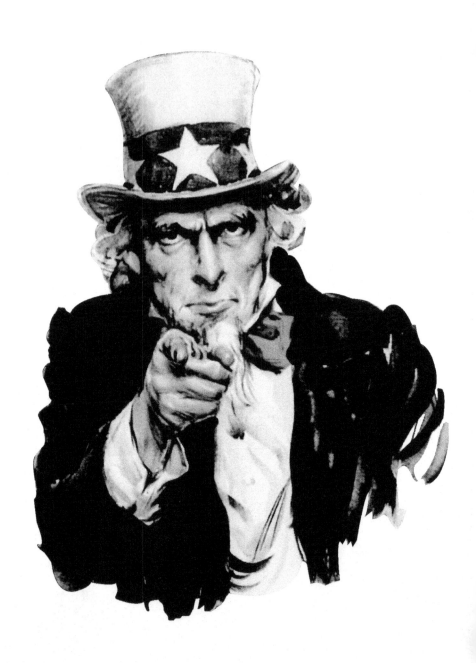

Degree Shift 31 – Your turn

YOU have now learned about carbohydrates, proteins, good fats, bad fats, Omega-3, Omega-6, soluble and insoluble fibre, glycaemic index, antioxidants, cholesterol, water consumption, food timing, portion size, coffee, tea and micronutrients. But what is knowledge if it is not used. What is knowing, without action? Can we hypothesise that too much knowledge without experience can cause confusion? Could we counter by saying a little bit of knowledge in the wrong hands can be worse than not knowing?

Let's put theory into practice. Let's really get some experience. What we have done over the past 30 lessons is give you the knowledge.

You have worked up to having the 'how' and the 'why,' so this time, let's put it all together by 'doing'. In fact, let's take it a step further by changing the 'doing' into 'teaching'. This time, we swap roles, and you become the teacher. There is a theory that the best way to really learn something is to teach it to someone else – preferably a crowd of people – imagine if you had to teach a million people...

You are going to take all your recently acquired knowledge and experience and put it together with one final nutritional experience... Practice, not theory. Through effect, we learn the cause. We cannot learn the effect through analysing a cause, because a cause by virtue of definition needs an effect. Without an effect, a cause is simply an idle thought – with infinite potential. Being fit and healthy does not come from knowing fit and healthy. It comes from the action, the doing fit and healthy things. Talking about being healthy isn't making you healthy, it's the actual act of doing healthy things that makes you a leader and an inspiration in the field of health and fitness. So here is your chance to do, and lock it in by teaching. Be inspirational!

You are going to design a meal that fits in with everything that we have learned, as well as your lifestyle. Put on your chef's hat, and get creative. Here are the rules of the game:

- Your meal must fit on a sideplate

- Your meal must have the following proportions:

  * Half fibrous carbohydrates

  * One quarter low fat protein source

  * One quarter (max) starchy carbohydrates

  * Sprinkling of good fats

- Your meal must taste delicious (if it doesn't, will you really eat it?)

- You must take a photograph of your meal, and send it to us with the completed form on the next page. Please send to the address at the front of this book.

- You must describe your meal, and how to prepare it.

Why stop at one meal? Why not make the whole week? Get creative, have fun – food is not boring. There are a million different variations you could come up with that are within the parameters. Now here is the fun part... if your recipe fits with all the rules, it will be used as one of the recipes in the *Never Diet Again* recipe book, and you will receive full credit as the creating chef.

Wouldn't that make you feel special? A healthy eating, glossy cookbook filled with only delicious healthy recipes, and on one page a recipe designed by you. With your name underneath it. Brag to everybody who wants to listen, because you are a contributor to a cookbook. (Unfortunately this eliminates plagiarising someone else's cook book of course!)

Chef's name: *(your name)*	
Meal name: *(be creative)*	
Photo attached *(circle):*	Yes / Yes[1]
Ingredients: *Fibrous Carbohydrates:* *Proteins:* *Starchy Carbohydrates:* *Fats:* *Flavouring / Seasoning:* *Other:*	

[1] There is only one option

Preparation instructions:

Why this meal is great:

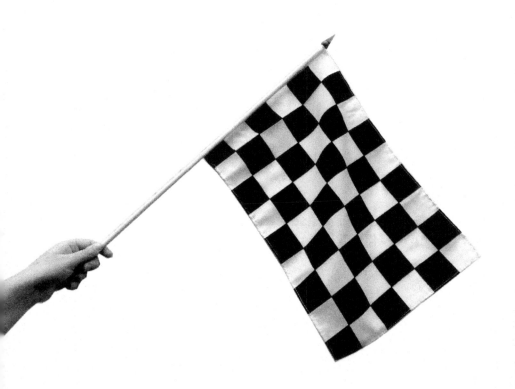

Degree Shift 32 - Conclusion

CONGRATULATIONS on completing your test for *Never Diet Again Part 2 – Food Quality*. **There is only one more** *Degree Shift* **that you need to discover to graduate. In creating your meal, you had to keep within the exact proportions of a perfect meal.**

Now the term perfect meal is used very loosely. The reason being that this should be your "go to" meal that you can adjust, depending on your body's needs. Keep in mind that the proportions that matter most are the totals for a full day, and you can adjust each individual meal's proportions depending on your energy needs for the day.

The first thing to think about is the overall energy expenditure in a 24 hour day. If you have a standard 8 hour sleep, this means you have 16 hours of awake time. We know that we use more energy being awake than asleep (needing carbohydrates), and that our bodies repair while we sleep (needing protein). Therefore, we can have:

- More starchy carbohydrate in the first 12 hours after waking

- More protein in the last meal of the day (in preparation for sleep)

Now examine where your exercise is timed for the day. Through exercise, you use up glycogen (stored carbohydrates), so the meal after exercise can include a higher proportion of starchy carbohydrates, without them being converted to fat. In fact, it has been well reported that your largest meal of the week should be eaten 1 – 3 hours after doing a resistance training session (assuming you only do one session per week).

If you were going to have simple carbohydrates, this is where you can have them, for least fat storage and higher muscle glycogen uptake. Levels vary for each person, but bodybuilders eat a set amount of simple carbohydrates immediately after strength training to replace glycogen, as well as to give them an insulin spike – which helps the uptake of protein to the muscles that are engorged with blood. But be careful – insulin stays in your system for up to 6 hours, meaning any excess carbohydrate or fat is stored as body fat.

Now take into consideration the need for antioxidants.

Essentially, they are needed at all times, but especially after exercise. Remember that exercise creates free radicals. Therefore, the meal after exercise could be lean steak (protein) with a salad (fibrous carbohydrates providing antioxidants) and virgin olive oil dressing or avocado (good fats). If it is the beginning of the day, we would require some starchy carbohydrates; you could add some brown rice (if you have had simple carbohydrates after your workout, then you won't need any here).

The point is that you should discover what is best for your body. We are all different. What proportions that work for you may be different to the proportions that work for someone else. Just remember the following:

- You should always have some carbohydrate, some protein and some fat in every meal. Just play with the proportions.

- This goes for breakfast as well. A western breakfast cereal diet means that we eat carbohydrates for breakfast, but often neglect protein. Along with the tissue building properties, protein helps you to feel full for longer. Remember too, that your body has had no protein since your last meal, yesterday.

- Try to keep all your meals the same size (except the one after resistance training)

If you stick to these guidelines, you will give your body the best chance of being a fat burning machine, as well as provide you with consistent energy levels throughout the day rather than the high / low of most people's current eating habits.

On behalf of your body, thank you so much for putting in the time to improve your food decisions through education and experience. You now belong to an elite group of people who can actually make their own decisions about foods, diets and nutrition from not only education, but experience. The greatest teacher of all.

Appendix 1: Hero to legend

THIS is to be read once you have completed your goal as set out in *Degree Shift 2*

Congratulations on completing your first life goal that you have set for yourself. The following is an excerpt from *Degree Shift 2*

"...your task is to create a tangible goal. Think of an event, one that you could have seen on TV, or heard about, or know of that requires physical endurance (fitness) to complete. Something that you "always wanted to do", something that you (or those around you) think is impossible in your current state."

It has to be something that you, or those around you don't think that you can do.

Later on, we realised that you were the only person who believed you could not achieve your goal. Take some time now to reflect on your achievement. Think about what you have done, and what it means to the people around you. You have completed an impossible challenge. You have climbed an insurmountable obstacle. You have defied belief. You are the destroyer of expectations. You are the commander of your destiny. You are a hero.

Heroes look at impossible tasks while others shy away and say: "I'll give it a go." Everybody else looks in awe and respect, as piece by piece, step by step, you – the hero – conquer your fear, throwing perceived restraints in the face of adversity and humbly conquering the unconquerable. You are true inspiration.

Now it is time to choose another task. Another impossible task. Make it big. Make it scary. You owe it to the people that you inspire. You owe it to yourself. When you die, what is it that you want to be remembered for?

Now is your chance to turn yourself from a hero into a legend.

My name is:	
My event is:	
The date my event is normally run:	
Who thinks I can't do it?	
Why I would like to do it:	

Appendix 2 – Answers to test

1. True

2. False

3. C

4. C

5. Polyunsaturated, Monounsaturated, Saturated, Trans

6. True

7. False

8. A

9. B

10. A

11. True

12. False

13. C

14. C

15. False

16. True

17. E

18. True

19. True

20. True

21. True

IMPORTANT!

BEFORE YOU BEGIN:

Go to:

www.sharnyandjulius.com/members

to register your copy of *Never Diet Again* and get INSTANT ACCESS to over $270 worth of FREE training.

About the Authors
Sharny and Julius

Renegade fitness experts Sharny and Julius shot to stardom very quickly when *Never Diet Again* was first released to the public in June 2011. The book was an adaptation of their step by step *escape the diet trap* program they created for their private clients. So successful was the program in changing people's lives that the clients literally begged Sharny and Julius to make it into a book, which would be more accessible to friends and relatives overseas.

After the release of *Never Diet Again*, the couple went on to write the book *FITlosophy*. In their words, it is "a collection of parables for athletes". But after consuming it, readers agree that it is far more than that. It is a profound set of philosophical viewpoints that cut right to the heart of the human condition.

Brutally honest, courageous, confronting, and often humorous, the stories told in this book reveal a part of the human psyche readers didn't even know was there. *FITlosophy* will sit with the reader for a long time after the words have actually been read.

For the release of *FITlosophy*, Sharny and Julius updated the cover of *Never Diet Again*, because they compliment each other perfectly. People who read Never Diet Again will naturally want to read *FITlosophy* and vice versa.

In January 2012, they collaborated with renowned artist Ayesha

Henderson to create a children's book that had "beautiful bright pictures and an easy to read, but important message that they could share with their kids". *Where Have All The Pixies Gone?* was released in October 2012.

At the time of publication, Sharny and Julius are writing the sequel to *FITlosophy*, which promises to be their magnum opus, their "greatest gift to humanity". They are regulars on daytime TV, radio and newspapers in their home country of Australia.

The couple are expecting their fourth child in January 2013 and plan on having one more. Sharny is the high energy super mum personality in the couple. Julius' often deep, philosophical nature is contrasted by his wicked sense of humour.

For more information or to contact Sharny and Julius, head to their private website\blog.

www.sharnyandjulius.com

Lightning Source UK Ltd.
Milton Keynes UK
UKOW05f0608230517
301817UK00012B/463/P